KARMA-YOGA

AND

BHAKTI-YOGA

RAMAKRISHNA-VIVEKANANDA CENTER
OF NEW YORK
17 East 94th Street, New York, N.Y. 10028

PUBLICATIONS

By Swami Nikhilananda

HINDUISM: Its Meaning for the Liberation of the Spirit

HOLY MOTHER: Being the Life of Sri Sarada Devi, Wife of Sri Ramakrishna and Helpmate in His Mission

MAN IN SEARCH OF IMMORTALITY: Testimonials from the Hindu Scriptures

VIVEKANANDA: A BIOGRAPHY

Translated by Swami Nikhilananda

THE BHAGAVAD GITA

THE BHAGAVAD GITA (Pocket Edition)

THE GOSPEL OF SRI RAMAKRISHNA

THE GOSPEL OF SRI RAMAKRISHNA (Abridged Edition)

SELF-KNOWLEDGE (Atmabodha)

THE UPANISHADS   Volumes I, II, III, and IV

By Swami Vivekananda

INSPIRED TALKS, My Master and Other Writings

JNANA-YOGA

KARMA-YOGA AND BHAKTI-YOGA

RAJA-YOGA

VIVEKANANDA: THE YOGAS AND OTHER WORKS
(Chosen and with a Biography by Swami Nikhilananda)

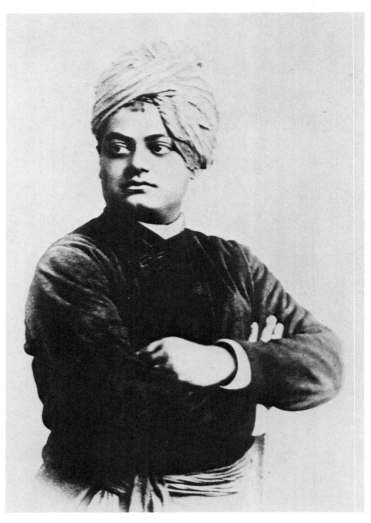

Vivekananda at the Parliament of Religions

KARMA-YOGA

AND

BHAKTI-YOGA

by

SWAMI VIVEKANANDA

REVISED EDITION

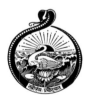

RAMAKRISHNA-VIVEKANANDA CENTER

NEW YORK

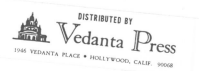

DISTRIBUTED BY

Vedanta Press

1946 VEDANTA PLACE • HOLLYWOOD, CALIF. 90068

PREFACE

The present revised edition of *Karma-Yoga and
Bhakti-Yoga* has been taken from *Vivekananda: The
Yogas and Other Works,* published in 1953 by the
Ramakrishna-Vivekananda Center of New York. The
following lines quoted from my preface to the latter
will explain the reasons for the editing of the book:
"Swami Vivekananda's public life covered a period
of ten years—from 1893, when he appeared at the
Parliament of Religions held in Chicago, to 1902,
when he gave up his mortal body. These were years
of great physical and mental strain as a result of
extensive travels, adaptation to new environments,
opposition from detractors both in his native land and
abroad, incessant public lectures and private instruction, a heavy correspondence, and the organizing of
the Ramakrishna Order in India. Hard work and
ascetic practices undermined his health. The Swami
thus had no time to revise his books, which either
were dictated by him or consisted of lectures delivered
without notes and taken down in shorthand or long-
hand. . . . I have therefore felt the need of editing
the present collection, making changes wherever
they were absolutely necessary, but being always
mindful to keep intact the Swami's basic thought."
Ninety pages of new material from the lectures of
Swami Vivekananda have been added to the present
volume in order to give the reader access to more

v

of the Swami's teachings and also to make the present volume uniform with the other three books of the series.

NIKHILANANDA

Ramakrishna-Vivekananda Center
New York
February 21, 1955

CONTENTS

Note on the Pronunciation of Sanskrit and Vernacular Words

a	has	the	sound	of	*o* in *come*.
ā	„	„	„	„	*a* in *far*.
e	„	„	„	„	*e* in *bed*.
i	„	„	„	„	*ee* in *feel*.
o	„	„	„	„	*o* in *note*.
u	„	„	„	„	*u* in *full*.
ai, ay	„	„	„	„	*oy* in *boy*.
au	„	„	„	„	*o* pronounced deep in the throat.
ch	„	„	„	„	*ch* in *church*.
ḍ	„	„	„	„	hard *d* (in English).
g	„	„	„	„	*g* in *god*.
jn	„	„	„	„	hard *gy* (in English).
ś	„	„	„	„	*sh* in *shut*.
th	„	„	„	„	*t-h* in *boat-house*.

sh may be pronounced as in English.
t and d are soft as in French.

Other consonants appearing in the transliterations may be pronounced as in English.

Diacritical marks have generally not been used in proper names belonging to recent times or in modern and well-known geographical names.

UNIFORM WITH THIS EDITION

Rāja-Yoga
Jnāna-Yoga

KARMA-YOGA

KARMA AND ITS EFFECT ON CHARACTER

THE WORD *karma* is derived from the Sanskrit *kri,* "to do." All action is karma. Technically this word also means the effects of actions. In connexion with metaphysics it sometimes means the effects of which our past actions were the causes. But in karma-yoga we have simply to do with the word *karma* as meaning work.

The goal of man is knowledge. That is the one great ideal placed before us by Eastern philosophy. Not pleasure, but knowledge, is the goal of man. Pleasure and happiness come to an end. It is a mistake to suppose that pleasure is the goal; the cause of all the miseries we have in the world is that men foolishly think pleasure to be the ideal to strive for. After a time a man finds that it is not happiness, but knowledge, towards which he is going, and that both pleasure and pain are great teachers, and that he learns as much from pain as from pleasure. As pleasure and pain pass before his soul, they leave upon it different pictures, and the result of these combined impressions is what is called a man's "character." If you take the character of any man, it really is but the aggregate of tendencies, the sum total of the inclinations of his mind; you will find that misery and happiness are equal factors in the formation of that character. Happiness and misery have an equal share in moulding character, and in some instances misery is a better teacher than happiness. Were one to study the great characters the world

has produced, I dare say it would be found, in the
vast majority of cases, that misery taught them more
than happiness, poverty taught them more than wealth,
blows brought out their inner fire more than praise.
Now knowledge, again, is inherent in man. No
knowledge comes from outside; it is all inside. What
we say a man "knows" should, in strict psychological
language, be what he discovers or unveils; what a
man "learns" is really what he discovers by taking the
cover off his own soul, which is a mine of infinite
knowledge. We say that Newton discovered gravitation. Was it sitting anywhere in a corner waiting for
him? It was in his own mind. The right time came
and he found it out. All the knowledge that the world
has ever received comes from the mind; the infinite
library of the universe is in your own mind. The
external world is simply the suggestion, the occasion,
which sets you to studying your own mind; but the
object of your study is always your own mind. The
falling of an apple gave the suggestion to Newton,
and he studied his own mind; he rearranged all the
previous links of thought in his mind and discovered a
new link among them, which we call the law of gravitation. It was not in the apple nor in anything in the
centre of the earth. All knowledge, therefore, secular
or spiritual, is in the human mind. In many cases it is
not discovered, but remains covered. When the covering is being slowly taken off we say that we are "learning," and the advance of knowledge is made by the
advance of this process of uncovering. The man from
whom this veil is being lifted is the knowing man;
the man upon whom it lies thick is ignorant; and the

man from whom it has entirely gone is all-knowing, omniscient. There have been omniscient men, and, I believe, there will be yet; there will be many of them in years to come. Like fire in a piece of flint, knowledge exists in the mind. Suggestion is the friction which brings it out. So with all our feelings and actions. Our tears and our smiles, our joys and our griefs, our weeping and our laughter, our curses and our blessings, our praises and our blamings—every one of these we shall find, if we calmly study our own selves, to have been brought out from within ourselves by so many blows. The result is what we are. All these blows taken together are called karma—work, action. Every mental and physical blow that is given to the soul, by which, as it were, fire is struck from it, and by which its own power and knowledge are discovered, is karma, using the word in its widest sense. Thus we are all doing karma all the time. I am talking to you: that is karma. You are listening: that is karma. We breathe: that is karma. We walk: that is karma. Everything we do, physical or mental, is karma, and it leaves its marks on us.

There are certain works which are, as it were, the aggregate, the sum total, of a large number of smaller works. If we stand near the seashore and hear the waves dashing against the shingle, we think it is a great noise. And yet we know that one wave is really composed of millions and millions of minute waves: Each one of these is making a noise, and yet we do not hear it; it is only when they become the big aggregate that we hear them. Similarly every pulsation of the heart is work. Certain kinds of work we feel and they become tangible to us; they are, at the same time, the aggregate of a number of small works. If you really want to judge the character of a man, do not look at his great performances. Every fool can act as a hero at one time or another. Watch a man do his most common actions; those are indeed the things which will tell you the real character of a great man. Great occasions rouse even the lowest of human beings to some kind of greatness; but he alone is the really great man whose character is great always, the same wherever he may be.

Karma in its effect on character is the most tremendous power that man has to deal with. Man is, as it were, a centre and is attracting all the powers of the universe towards himself, and in this centre is fusing them all and again sending them off in a big current. Such a centre is the real man, the almighty and the omniscient. He draws the whole universe towards him; good and bad, misery and happiness, all are running towards him and clinging round him. And out of them he fashions the mighty stream of tendency called character and throws it outwards. As he has the power of drawing in anything, so has he the power of throwing it out.

All the actions that we see in the world, all the movements in human society, all the works that we have around us, are simply the display of thought, the manifestation of the will of man. Machines, instruments, cities, ships, men-of-war—all these are simply the manifestation of the will of man; and this will is caused by character, and character is manufactured from karma. As is the karma, so is the manifestation of the will. The men of mighty will the world has produced have all been tremendous workers—gigantic souls with wills powerful enough to overturn worlds, wills they got by persistent work through ages and ages. Such a gigantic will as that of a Buddha or a Jesus could not be obtained in one life, for we know who their fathers were. It is not known that their fathers ever spoke a word for the good of mankind. Millions and millions of carpenters like Joseph had come and gone; millions are still living. Millions and millions of petty kings like Buddha's father had been in the world. If it was only a case of hereditary transmission, how do you account for the fact that this petty prince, who was not, perhaps, obeyed by his own servants, produced a son whom half the world worships? How do you explain the gulf between the carpenter and his son, whom millions of human beings worship as God? It cannot be solved by the theory of heredity. The gigantic will which manifested Buddha and Jesus —whence did it come? Whence came this accumulation of power? It must have been there through ages and ages, continually growing bigger and bigger until it burst on society as Buddha or Jesus, and it is rolling down even to the present day.

All this is determined by karma, work. No one can get anything unless he earns it; this is an eternal law. We may sometimes think it is not so, but in the long run we become convinced of it. A man may struggle all his life for riches; he may cheat thousands; but he finds at last that he does not deserve to become rich and his life becomes a trouble and a nuisance to him.

We may go on accumulating things for our physical enjoyment, but only what we earn is really ours. A fool may buy all the books in the world, and they will be in his library; but he will be able to read only those that he deserves to. This deserving is produced by karma. Our karma determines what we deserve and what we can assimilate. We are responsible for what we are; and whatever we wish ourselves to be, we have the power to make ourselves. If what we are now has been the result of our own past actions, it certainly follows that whatever we wish to be in the future can be produced by our present actions. So we have to know how to act. You will say: "What is the use of learning how to work? Everyone works in some way or other in this world." But there is such a thing as frittering away our energies. Karma-yoga, the Bhagavad Gītā says, is doing work with cleverness and as a science. By knowing how to work one can obtain the greatest results. You must remember that the aim of all work is simply to bring out the power of the mind which is already there, to wake up the soul. The power is inside every man; and so is knowledge. Different works are like blows to bring them out, to cause these giants to wake up.

Man works with various motives; there cannot be work without motive. Some people want to get fame and they work for fame. Others want money and they work for money. Some want to have power and they work for power. Others want to get to heaven and they work for that. Still others want to earn a name for their ancestors, as in China, where no man gets a title until he is dead; and that is a better way, after all, than ours. When a man does something very good there, they give a title of nobility to his dead father or grandfather. Some people work for that. Some of the followers of certain Mohammedan sects work all their lives to have a big tomb built for them when they die. I know sects among whom, as soon as a child is born, a tomb is started; that is among them the most important work a man has to do; and the bigger and the finer the tomb, the happier the man is supposed to be. Others work as a penance; they do all sorts of wicked things and then erect a temple or give something to the priests to buy them off and obtain a passport to heaven. They think that this kind of beneficence will clear them and that they will go scot-free in spite of their sinfulness. Such are some of the various motives for work.

Now let us consider work for work's sake. There are some who are really the salt of the earth, who work for work's sake, who do not care for name or fame or even to go to heaven. They work just because good will come of it. There are others who do good to the poor and help mankind from still higher motives, because they believe in doing good and they love good. As a rule, the desire for name and fame seldom brings quick results; they come to us when we are old and have almost done with life. If a man works without any selfish motive, does he not gain something? Yes, he gains the highest benefit. Unselfishness is more paying; only people have not the patience to practise it. It is more paying from the point of view of health also. Love, truth, and unselfishness are not merely figures of speech used by moralists, but they form our

highest ideal, because in them lies such a manifestation
of power. In the first place, a man who can work for
five days, or even five minutes, without any selfish
motive whatever, without thinking of the future, of
heaven, of punishment, or anything of the kind, has
in him the capacity to become a powerful moral giant.
It is hard to do it, but in our heart of hearts we know
its value and the good it brings.

It is the greatest manifestation of power, this tremendous restraint; self-restraint is a manifestation of
greater power than any selfish action. A carriage with
four horses may rush down a hill unrestrained, or the
coachman may curb the horses. Which is the greater
display of power—to let the horses go or to hold them?
A cannon-ball flying through the air goes a long distance and falls. Another is cut short in its flight by
striking against a wall, and the impact generates intense heat. All outgoing energy following from a selfish motive is frittered away; it will not cause power to
return to you; but if selfishness is restrained, it will
result in the development of power. This self-control
will tend to produce a mighty will, a character which
makes a Christ or a Buddha. Foolish men do not know
this secret; they nevertheless want to rule mankind.
Even a fool may rule the whole world if he works and
waits. Let him wait a few years, restrain that foolish
idea of governing, and when that idea is wholly gone,
he will be a power in the world. The majority of us
cannot see beyond a few years, as some animals cannot see beyond a few steps. Just a little narrow circle
—that is our world. We have not the patience to look

beyond, and thus we become immoral and wicked. This is our weakness, our powerlessness. Even the lowest forms of work are not to be despised. Let the man who knows no better work for selfish ends, for name and fame; but everyone should always try to move towards higher and higher motives and to understand them. "To work we have the right, but not to the fruits thereof." Leave the fruits alone. Why care for results? If you wish to help a man, never think what that man's attitude should be towards you. If you want to do a great or a good work, do not trouble to think what the result will be.

There arises a difficult question in this ideal of work. Intense activity is necessary; we must always work. We cannot live a minute without work. What then becomes of rest? Here is one side of life: struggle and work by which we are whirled rapidly round. And here is the other: calm, retiring renunciation—everything is peaceful around, there is very little of noise and show, only nature with her animals and flowers and mountains. Neither of them is a perfect picture. A man used to solitude, if brought in contact with the surging whirlpool of the world, will be crushed by it, just as the fish that lives in deep-sea water, as soon as it is brought to the surface, breaks into pieces, deprived of the weight of water on it that kept it together. Can a man who has been used to the turmoil and the rush of life live at ease if he comes to a quiet place? He suffers and perchance may lose his mind. The ideal man is he who in the midst of the greatest silence and solitude finds the intensest activity, and in the midst of the intensest activity, the silence and solitude of the desert. He has learnt the secret of restraint; he has controlled himself. He goes through the streets of a big city with all its traffic, and his mind is calm as if he were in a cave where not a sound could reach him; but he is intensely working all the time. That is the ideal of karma-yoga; and if you have attained to that you have really learnt the secret of work.

But we have to start from the beginning, to take up works as they come to us and slowly make ourselves more unselfish every day. We must do the work and find out the motive that prompts us; and in the first years we shall find that almost without exception our motives are selfish. But gradually this selfishness will melt through persistence, and at last will come the time when we shall be able to do really unselfish work. We may all hope that some day or other, as we struggle through the paths of life, there will come a time when we shall become perfectly unselfish; and the moment we attain to that, all our powers will be concentrated and the knowledge which is ours will be manifest.

EACH IS GREAT IN HIS OWN PLACE

ACCORDING TO THE Sāmkhya philosophy, nature is composed of three forces called, in Sanskrit, sattva, rajas, and tamas. These, as manifested in the physical world, are what we may call equilibrium, activity, and inertness. Tamas typifies darkness or inactivity; rajas is activity, expressed as attraction or repulsion; and sattva is the equilibrium of the two. In every man there are these three forces. Sometimes tamas prevails and we become lazy, we cannot move; we are inactive, bound down by certain set ideas or by mere dullness. At other times activity prevails, and at still other times the calm balancing of both. Again, in different men, one of these forces is generally predominant. The characteristic of one man is inactivity, dullness, and laziness; that of another, activity, power, manifestation of energy; and in still another we find sweetness, calmness, and gentleness, which are due to the balancing of both action and inaction. So in all created beings—in animals, plants, and men— we find more or less typical manifestations of these different forces. Karma-yoga has especially to deal with these three factors. By teaching what they are and how to employ them it helps us to do our work better.

Human society is a graded organization. We all know about morality and we all know about duty, but at the same time we find that in different countries the significance of morality varies greatly. What is regarded as moral in one country may in another be

13

considered perfectly immoral. For instance, in one country cousins may marry; in another this is thought to be very immoral; in one, men may marry their sisters-in-law; in another, that is regarded as immoral; in one country people may have only one wife; in another, many wives; and so forth. Similarly, in all other departments of morality we find that the standard varies greatly; yet we feel that there must be a universal standard of morality.

So it is with duty. The idea of duty varies much among different nations. In one country, if a man does not do certain things, people will say he has acted wrongly, while in another country, if he does those very things, people will say he has acted wrongly; and yet we know that there must be some universal idea of duty. In the same way, one class of society thinks that certain things are among its duties, while another class thinks quite the opposite and would be horrified if it had to do those things. Two ways are left open to us: the way of the ignorant, who think that there is only one way to truth and that all the rest are wrong; and the way of the wise, who admit that, according to our mental constitution or the different circumstances in which we dwell, duty and morality may vary. The important thing is to know that there are gradations of duty and of morality—that the duty of one state of life, in one set of circumstances, will not and cannot be that of another.

For example, all great teachers have taught: "Resist not evil"—that non-resistance is the highest moral ideal. But we also know that if even a small number of us tried to put that maxim fully into practice, the whole social fabric would fall to pieces, the wicked would take possession of our properties and our lives, and would do whatever they liked with us. Even if for only one day such non-resistance were practised it would lead to disaster. Yet intuitively, in our heart of hearts, we feel the truth of the teaching, "Resist not evil." This seems to us to be the highest ideal; yet to teach only this doctrine would be equivalent to condemning a vast portion of mankind. Not only so; it would make many feel that they were always doing wrong, cause in them scruples of conscience in all their actions; it would weaken them, and that constant self-disapproval would breed more vice than any other weakness would. To the man who has begun to hate himself, the gate to degeneration has already opened; and the same is true of a nation. Our first duty is not to hate ourselves; to advance we must have faith in ourselves first and then in God. He who has no faith in himself can never have faith in God. Therefore the only alternative remaining to us is to recognize that duty and morality vary under different circumstances. The man who resists evil is not necessarily doing what is always and in itself wrong, but under the circumstances in which he is placed it may even become his duty to resist evil.

In reading the Bhagavad Gītā, many of you in Western countries may have felt astonished at the second chapter, wherein, when Arjuna refuses to fight or offer resistance, because his adversaries are his friends and relatives, and makes the plea that non-resistance is the highest ideal of love, Śri Krishna calls him a hypocrite and a coward. There is a great lesson

for us all to learn—that in all matters the two extremes are alike. The extreme positive and the extreme
negative are always similar. When the vibrations of
light are too low we do not see them, nor do we see
them when they are too intense. So with sound: when
it is very low in pitch we do not hear it, when very
high we do not hear it either. Of like nature is the
difference between resistance and non-resistance. One
man does not resist because he is weak and lazy, and
he will not because he cannot; the other man knows
that he can strike an irresistible blow if he likes; yet
he not only does not strike, but blesses his enemies.
The one who from weakness resists not commits a
sin and hence cannot receive any benefit from the non-
resistance; while the other would commit a sin by
offering resistance. Buddha gave up his throne and
renounced his position; that was true renunciation.
But there cannot be any question of renunciation in
the case of a beggar who has nothing to renounce. So
we must always be careful about what we really mean
when we speak of non-resistance and ideal love. We
must first take care to understand whether we have
the power of resistance or not. Then, having the
power, if we renounce it and do not resist, we are
doing a grand act of love; but if we cannot resist, and
yet, at the same time, try to deceive ourselves into the
belief that we are actuated by motives of the highest
love, we are doing the exact opposite. Arjuna became
a coward at the sight of the mighty array against him;
his "love" made him forget his duty towards his country and king. That is why Śri Krishna told him that
he was a hypocrite: "Thou talkest like a wise man,

but thy actions betray thee to be a coward; therefore stand up and fight!"

Such is the central idea of karma-yoga. The karma-yogi is the man who understands that the highest ideal is non-resistance, and who also knows that this non-resistance is the highest manifestation of power; but he knows, too, that what is called the resisting of evil is a step on the way towards the manifestation of this highest power, namely, non-resistance. Before reaching this highest ideal man's duty is to resist evil. Let him work, let him fight, let him strike straight from the shoulder. Then only, when he has gained the power to resist, will non-resistance be a virtue.

I once met a man in my country whom I had known before as a very stupid, dull person, who knew nothing and had not the desire to know anything and was living the life of a brute. He asked me what he should do to know God, how he was to get free. "Can you tell a lie?" I asked him. "No," he replied. "Then you must learn to do so. It is better to tell a lie than to be a brute or a log of wood. You are inactive; you have certainly not reached the highest state, which is beyond all action, calm and serene. You are too dull even to do something wicked." That was an extreme case, of course, and I was joking with him; but what I meant was that a man must be active in order to pass through activity to perfect calmness. Inactivity should be avoided by all means. Activity always means resistance. Resist all evils, mental and physical; and when you have succeeded in resisting, then calmness will come.

It is very easy to say, "Hate nobody, resist not evil,"

but we know what that kind of advice generally means in practice. When the eyes of society are turned towards us we may make a show of non-resistance, but in our hearts there is canker all the time. We feel the utter want of the calm of non-resistance; we feel that it would be better for us to resist. Further, if you desire wealth, and know at the same time that the whole world regards him who aims at wealth as a very wicked man, you will perhaps not dare to plunge into the struggle for wealth; yet your mind will be running day and night after money. This is hypocrisy and will serve no purpose. Plunge into the world, and then, after a time, when you have suffered and enjoyed all that is in it, will renunciation come, then will calmness come. So fulfil your desire for power and everything else; and after you have fulfilled the desire, will come the time when you shall know that they are all very little things. But until you have fulfilled this desire, until you have passed through that activity, it is impossible for you to come to the state of calmness, serenity, and self-surrender. These ideas of serenity and renunciation have been preached for thousands of years; everybody has heard of them from childhood; and yet we see very few in the world who have really realized them. I do not know if I have seen twenty persons in my life who are really calm and non-resisting, and I have travelled over half the world.

Every man should take up his own ideal and endeavour to accomplish it; that is a surer way of progressing than taking up other men's ideals, which he can never hope to accomplish. For instance, we take a child and at once give him the task of walking twenty miles; either the little one dies or one in a thousand crawls the twenty miles to reach the end exhausted and half dead. That is what we generally try to do with the world. Not all the men and women in any society are of the same mind, capacity, or power to do things; they must have different ideals, and we have no right to sneer at any ideal. Let everyone do the best he can to realize his own ideal. Nor is it right that I should be judged by your standard or you by mine. The apple tree should not be judged by the standard of the oak, nor the oak by that of the apple. To judge the apple tree you must take the apple standard; and to judge the oak, its own standard.

Unity in variety is the plan of creation. However men and women may vary individually, there is unity in the background. The different individual characters and classes of men and women are natural variations in creation. Hence we ought not to judge them by the same standard or put the same ideal before them. Such a course only creates an unnatural struggle, and the result is that a man begins to hate himself and is hindered from becoming religious and good. Our duty is to encourage everyone in his struggle to live up to his own highest ideal, and strive at the same time to make that ideal as near as possible to the truth.

In the Hindu system of morality we find that this fact has been recognized from very ancient times; and in the Hindu scriptures and books on ethics different rules are laid down for the different classes of men—the student, the householder, the vānaprasthin, and the sannyāsin.

The life of every individual, according to the Hindu scriptures, has its peculiar duties apart from those which are common to humanity. The Hindu begins life as a student; then he marries and becomes a householder; in old age he retires; and lastly he gives up the world and becomes a sannyāsin. To each of these stages of life certain duties are attached. One of these stages is not intrinsically superior to another; the life of the married man is quite as great as that of the celibate who has devoted himself to religious work. The scavenger in the street is quite as great and glorious as the king on his throne. Take the king off his throne, make him do the scavenger's work, and see how he fares. Put the scavenger on the throne and see how he rules. It is useless to say that the man who lives outside the world is a greater man than he who lives in the world; it is much more difficult to live in the world and worship God than to give it up and live a free and easy life. The four stages of life in India have in later times been reduced to two: the life of the householder and that of the monk. The householder marries and carries on his duties as a citizen; the duty of the other is to devote his energies wholly to religion, to preach and to worship God. I shall present to you a few ideas from the *Mahānirvāna Tantra* which treat of this subject, and you will see that it is a very difficult task for a man to be a householder and perform all his duties perfectly:

The householder should be devoted to God; knowledge of God should be the goal of his life. Yet he must work constantly, perform all his duties; he must give up the fruits of his actions to God.

It is the most difficult thing in this world to work and not care for the result, to help a man and never think that he ought to be grateful, to do good work and at the same time never look back to see whether it brings you name or fame or nothing at all. Even the most arrant coward becomes brave when the world praises him. A fool can do heroic deeds when he receives the approbation of society; but to constantly do good without caring for the approbation of his fellow men is indeed the highest sacrifice a man can perform.

The great duty of the householder is to earn a living, but he must take care that he does not do it by telling lies or by cheating or by robbing others; and he must remember that his life is for the service of God and the poor.

Knowing that his mother and father are the visible representatives of God, the householder always and by all possible means must please them. If his mother is pleased, and his father, then God is pleased with that man. That child is really a good child who never speaks harsh words to his parents. Before one's parents one must not utter jokes, must not show restlessness, must not show anger or temper. Before his mother or father a child must bow down low; he must stand up in their presence and must not take a seat until they order him to sit.

If the householder enjoys food and drink and clothes without first seeing that his mother and father, his children, his wife, and the poor are supplied with them, he is committing a sin. The mother and father are the causes of this body; so a man must undergo a thousand troubles in order to do good to them.

Even so is his duty to his wife. No man should scold his wife, and he must always maintain her as if she were his own mother. And even when he is in the greatest difficulties and troubles, he must not renounce his wife if she is chaste and devoted to him.

He who cherishes another woman besides his wife —if he touches her even with his mind, that man goes to a dark hell.

Before women a man must not use improper language, and must never brag of his powers. He must not say, "I have done this, and I have done that."

The householder must always please his wife with money, clothes, love, faith, and words like nectar, and must never do anything to disturb her. That man who has succeeded in getting the love of a chaste wife has succeeded in his religion and has all the virtues.

The following are a man's duties towards his children:

A son should be lovingly reared up to his fourth year; he should be educated till he is sixteen. When he is twenty years of age he should be employed in some work; he should then be treated affectionately by his father as his equal. Exactly in the same manner the daughter should be brought up, and she should be educated with the greatest care. When she marries, the father ought to give her jewels and wealth.

Then there is the duty of a man towards his

brothers and sisters, and towards the children of his brothers and sisters, if they are poor, and towards his other relatives, his friends, and his servants. Further, there are his duties towards the people of the same village, and the poor, and anyone that comes to him for help. If the householder, having sufficient means, does not care to help his relatives and the poor, know him to be only a brute; he is not a human being.

Excessive attachment to food, clothes, and the tending of the body and the dressing of the hair should be avoided. The householder must be pure in heart and clean in body, always active and always ready for work.

To his enemies the householder must be a hero. When threatened by them he must resist. That is the duty of the householder. He must not sit down in a corner and weep, and talk nonsense about non-resistance. If he does not show himself a hero to his enemies, he has not done his duty. And to his friends and relatives he must be as gentle as a lamb.

It is the duty of the householder not to pay reverence to the wicked, because if he reverences the wicked people of the world, he patronizes wickedness. And it will be a great mistake if he disregards those who are worthy of respect, the good people. He must not be gushing in his friendship; he must not go out of his way to make friends everywhere; he must watch the actions of the men he wants to make friends with, and their dealings with other men, reflect upon them, and then make friends.

These three things he must not talk of: He must not talk in public of his own fame, or preach his

own name or his own powers; he must not talk of his
wealth; and he must not talk of anything that has
been told him privately.

A man must not say that he is poor or that he is
wealthy; he must not brag of his wealth. Let him
keep his own counsel; this is his religious duty. This
is not mere worldly wisdom; if a man does not do
so, he may be held to be immoral.

The householder is the basis, the prop, of the
whole of society; he is the principal earner. The
poor, the weak, and the women and children, who
do not work—all live upon the householder. So he
has certain duties towards them, and these duties
should be such as to make him feel strong while
performing them, and not make him think that he
is doing things beneath his ideal. Therefore if he has
done something unworthy or has made some mistake,
he must not say so in public; and if he is engaged in
some enterprise and knows he is sure to fail in it, he
must not speak of it. Such self-exposure is not only
uncalled for but also unnerves the man and makes
him unfit for the performance of his legitimate duties
in life. At the same time, he must struggle hard to
acquire two things: first, knowledge, and second,
wealth. This is his duty, and if he does not do his
duty he is nobody. A householder who does not
struggle to get wealth is immoral. If he is lazy and
content to lead an idle life, he is immoral, because
upon him depend hundreds. If he gets riches, hundreds of others will be thereby supported.

If there were not in this city hundreds who had
striven to become rich, and who had acquired wealth,

where would all this civilization and these almshouses and mansions be? Going after wealth in such a case is not bad, because that wealth is for distribution. The householder is the centre of life and society. It is a kind of worship for him to acquire and spend wealth nobly; for the householder who struggles to become rich by good means and for good purposes is doing practically the same thing for the attainment of salvation as the anchorite does in his cell when he prays; for in them we see only different aspects of the same virtue of self-surrender and self-sacrifice prompted by the feeling of devotion to God and to all that is His.

The householder must struggle to acquire a good name; he must not gamble; he must not move in the company of the wicked; he must not tell lies and must not be the cause of trouble to others.

Often people enter into things they have not the means to accomplish, with the result that they cheat others to attain their own ends. Then there is in all things the time factor to be taken into consideration; what at one time might be a failure would perhaps at another time be a very great success.

The calm householder must speak the truth and speak gently, using words which people like, which will do good to others; and he should not boast about himself or criticize other men.

The householder, by digging wells, by planting trees along the roadsides, by establishing rest-houses for men and animals, by making roads and building bridges, goes towards the same goal that the greatest yogi attains.

This is one part of the doctrine of karma-yoga—activity, the duty of the householder. There is a passage later on where the *Mahānirvāna Tantra* says: "If the householder dies in battle, fighting for his country or his religion, he comes to the same goal that the yogi attains through meditation," showing thereby that what is duty for one is not duty for another. At the same time, it does not say that the former duty is lowering, and the latter, elevating; each duty has its own place, and according to the circumstances in which we are placed must we perform our duties.

One idea comes out of all this: the condemnation of all weakness. This is a particular idea in all our teachings which I like, whether in philosophy or in religion or in work. If you read the Vedas you will find one word always repeated: "fearlessness." Fear nothing. Fear is a sign of weakness. A man must go about his duties without taking notice of the sneers and the ridicule of the world.

If a man retires from the world to worship God, he must not think that those who live in the world and work for the good of the world are not worshipping God. Neither must those who live in the world, working for the good of wife and children, think that those who give up the world are low vagabonds. Each is great in his own place. This thought I will illustrate by a story.

A certain king used to inquire of all the sannyāsins that came to his country, "Which is the greater man—he who gives up the world and becomes a sannyāsin or he who lives in the world and performs his duties as a householder?" Many wise monks sought to solve the problem. Some asserted that the sannyāsin was the greater, upon which the king demanded that they prove their assertion. When they could not do so, he ordered them to marry and become householders. Then others came and said, "The householder who performs his duties is the greater man." Of them, too, the king demanded proofs. When they could not give them, he made them also settle down as householders.

At last there came a young sannyāsin, and the king asked him the same question. He said, "Each, O King, is great in his own place." "Prove this to me," demanded the king. "I will prove it to you," said the sannyāsin, "but you must come and live with me for a few days, that I may be able to prove to you what I say." The king consented. He followed the sannyāsin out of his own territory and they passed through many other countries until they came to a great kingdom. In the capital of that kingdom a ceremony was going on. The king and the sannyāsin heard the noise of drums and music, and heard also the criers; the people were assembled in the streets in gala dress, and a proclamation was being made. The king and the sannyāsin stood there to see what was going on. The crier was proclaiming loudly that the princess, daughter of the king of that country, was about to choose a husband from among those assembled before her.

It was an old custom in India for princesses to choose husbands in this way. Each princess had certain ideas of the sort of man she wanted for a hus-

band. Some wanted the handsomest man, others
wanted only the most learned, others again the rich-
est, and so on. All the princes of the neighbourhood
would put on their best attire and present themselves
before her. Sometimes they too had their own criers
to enumerate their virtues—the reasons why they
hoped the princess would choose them. The princess
would be taken round on a throne, in the most splendid array, and would look at them and hear about
them. If she was not pleased with what she saw and
heard, she would say to her bearers, "Move on," and
would take no more notice of the rejected suitor. If,
however, the princess was pleased with any one of
them, she would throw a garland of flowers over
him and he became her husband.

The princess of the country to which our king
and the sannyāsin had come was having one of these
interesting ceremonies. She was the most beautiful
princess in the world, and her husband would be
ruler of the kingdom after her father's death. The
idea of this princess was to marry the handsomest
man, but she could not find one to please her. Several
such meetings had taken place, but the princess had
been unable to select a husband. This meeting was
the most splendid of all; more people than ever before
attended it. The princess came in on a throne, and
the bearers carried her from place to place. She did
not seem to care for anyone, and everyone was dis-
appointed, thinking that this meeting also was going
to be a failure.

Just then a young man, a sannyāsin, radiant as if
the sun had come down to the earth, came and stood

in one corner of the assembly, watching what was going on. The throne with the princess came near him, and as soon as she saw the beautiful sannyāsin, she stopped and threw the garland over him. The young sannyāsin seized the garland and threw it off, exclaiming: "What nonsense is this? I am a sannyāsin. What is marriage to me?" The king of that country thought that perhaps this man was poor and so dared not marry the princess, and said to him, "With my daughter goes half my kingdom now, and the whole kingdom after my death!" and put the garland on the sannyāsin again. The young man threw it off once more, saying, "Nonsense! I do not want to marry," and walked quickly away from the assembly.

Now, the princess had fallen so much in love with this young man that she said, "I must marry this man or I shall die"; and she went after him to bring him back. Then our other sannyāsin, who had brought the king there, said to him, "King, let us follow this pair." So they went after them, but at a good distance behind. The young sannyāsin who had refused to marry the princess walked out into the country for several miles. When he came to a forest and entered it, the princess followed him, and the other two followed also. Now this young sannyāsin was well acquainted with that forest and knew all the intricate paths in it. He suddenly entered one of these and disappeared, and the princess could not discover him. After vainly trying for a long time to find him, she sat down under a tree and began to weep, for she did not know the way out. Then our king and the other sannyāsin came up to her and said: "Do not weep. We shall show you the way out of this forest, but it is too dark for us to find it now. Here is a big tree; let us rest under it, and in the morning we shall show you the road."

Now, a little bird and his wife and their three young ones lived in that tree, in a nest. This little bird looked down and saw the people under the tree and said to his wife: "My dear, what shall we do? Here are some guests in the house, and it is winter, and we have no fire." So he flew away and got a bit of burning firewood in his beak and dropped it before the guests, to which they added fuel and made a blazing fire. But the little bird was not satisfied. He said again to his wife: "My dear, what shall we do? There is nothing to give these people to eat, and they are hungry. We are householders; it is our duty to feed anyone who comes to the house. I must do what I can; I will give them my body." So he plunged into the fire and perished. The guests saw him falling and tried to save him, but he was too quick for them.

The little bird's wife saw what her husband did, and she said: "Here are three persons and there is only one little bird for them to eat. It is not enough; it is my duty as a wife not to let my husband's efforts go in vain. Let them have my body also." Then she fell into the fire and was burnt to death.

Then the three baby birds, when they saw what was done and that there was still not enough food for the three guests, said: "Our parents have done what they could and still it is not enough. It is our duty to carry on the work of our parents. Let our bodies go." And they too dashed down into the fire. Amazed at what they saw, the three people could not of course eat these birds. They passed the night without food, and in the morning the king and the sannyāsin showed the princess the way, and she went back to her father.

Then the sannyāsin said to the king: "King, you have seen that each is great in his own place. If you want to live in the world, live like those birds, ready at any moment to sacrifice yourself for others. If you want to renounce the world, be like that young man, to whom the most beautiful woman and a kingdom were as nothing. If you want to be a householder, hold your life as a sacrifice for the welfare of others; and if you choose the life of renunciation, do not even look at beauty and money and power. Each is great in his own place, but the duty of the one is not the duty of the other."

THE SECRET OF WORK

HELPING OTHERS physically, by removing their physical needs, is indeed great; but the help is greater according as the need is greater and the help more far-reaching. If a man's wants can be removed for an hour, it is helping him indeed; if his wants can be removed for a year, it will be rendering him more help; but if his wants can be removed for ever, it is surely the greatest help that can be given him.

Spiritual knowledge is the only thing that can destroy our miseries for ever; any other knowledge removes wants only for a time. It is only with the knowledge of the Spirit that the root cause of want is destroyed for ever; so helping man spiritually is the highest help that can be given him. He who gives man spiritual knowledge is the greatest benefactor of mankind, and we always find that they are the most powerful who help man in his spiritual needs, because spirituality is the true inspiration of all our activities. A spiritually strong and sound man will be strong in every other respect, if he so wishes. Until there is spiritual strength in a man, even physical needs cannot be well satisfied.

Next to spiritual comes intellectual help. The gift of knowledge is a far higher gift than that of food and clothes; it is even higher than giving life to a man, because the real life of man consists in knowledge. Ignorance is death; knowledge is life. Life is of very little value if it is a life in the dark, groping through ignorance and misery.

Next in order comes, of course, helping a man physically. Therefore, in considering the question of helping others, we must always strive not to commit the mistake of thinking that physical help is the only help that can be given. It is not only the last but the least, because it cannot give any permanent satisfaction. The misery that I feel when I am hungry is satisfied by eating, but hunger returns; my misery can cease for ever only when I am beyond all physical wants. Then hunger will not make me miserable; no distress, no sorrow, will be able to move me. So that help which tends to make us strong spiritually is the highest, next to it comes intellectual help, and after that physical help.

The miseries of the world cannot be cured by physical help only; until a man's nature changes, these physical needs will always arise and miseries will always be felt, and no amount of physical help will cure them completely. The only lasting solution is to give man spiritual wisdom. Ignorance is the mother of all the evil and all the misery we see. Let men have light, let them be pure and spiritually strong and educated; then alone will misery cease in the world, and not before. We may convert every house in the country into a charity asylum; we may fill the land with hospitals; but the misery of man will continue to exist until man's character changes.

We read in the Bhagavad Gītā again and again that we must all work incessantly. All work is by nature composed of good and evil. We cannot do any

work which will not do some good somewhere; there
cannot be any work which will not cause some harm
somewhere. Every work must necessarily be a mixture of good and evil. Yet we are commanded to work
incessantly. Good and evil will both have their results, will bear their fruit. Good action will produce
good effects; bad action, bad. But good and bad are
both bondages of the soul. The solution reached in
the Gitā in regard to the bondage-producing nature
of work is that if we do not attach ourselves to the
work we do, it will not have any binding effect on
our soul. This is the one central idea in the Gitā:
work incessantly, but be not attached. We shall try
to understand what is meant by non-attachment to
work.

The word *samskāra* can be translated very nearly
by "inherent tendency." To use the simile of a lake
for the mind: a ripple or a wave that rises in the
mind does not die out entirely when it subsides, but
leaves a mark and a future possibility of its coming
back. This mark, with the possibility of the wave's
reappearing, is what is called a samskāra.

Every work we do, every movement of our body,
every thought we think, leaves such an impression
on the mind-stuff; and even when these impressions
are not obvious on the surface, they are sufficiently
strong to work beneath the surface, subconsciously.
What we are at every moment is determined by the
sum total of these impressions in the mind. What I
am just at this moment is the effect of the sum total
of all the impressions of my past. This is really what
is meant by character; each man's character is de-

termined by the sum total of these impressions. If good impressions prevail, the character becomes good; if bad, it becomes bad. If a man continually hears bad words, thinks bad thoughts, does bad deeds, his mind will be full of bad impressions; and they will influence his thought and work without his being conscious of the fact. These bad impressions are always working, and their resultant must be evil; and that man will be a bad man; he cannot help it. The sum total of these impressions in him will create a strong motive power for doing bad deeds; he will be like a tool in the hands of his impressions, and they will force him to do evil. Similarly, if a man thinks good thoughts and does good works, the sum total of these impressions will be good; and they, in a similar manner, will force him to do good even in spite of himself. When a man has done much good work and thought many good thoughts, there is created in him an irresistible tendency to do good. His mind, controlled by the sum total of his good tendencies, will not then allow him to do evil even if he wishes to do so. The tendencies will turn him back; he is completely under the influence of the good tendencies. When such is the case, a man's good character is said to be established.

When the tortoise tucks its head and feet inside its shell, you may kill it and break the shell to pieces, and yet the head and feet will not come out; even so the character of that man who has control over his motives and organs is unchangeably established. He controls his own inner forces, and nothing can draw them out against his will. Through the continuous reflex action of good thoughts and good impressions moving over the surface of the mind, the tendency for doing good becomes strong, and as a result we feel able to control the indriyas—the sense-organs, the nerve-centres. Thus alone is character established; then alone does a man attain to truth. Such a man is safe for ever; he cannot do any evil. You may place him in any company; there will be no danger for him.

There is a still higher state than having this good tendency, and that is the desire for liberation. You must remember that freedom of the soul is the goal of all the yogas, and all of them lead to the same result. By work alone men may get to where Buddha got largely by meditation or Christ by prayer. Buddha was a working jnāni; Christ was a bhakta; but the same goal was reached by both of them. The difficulty is here: Liberation means entire freedom—freedom from the bondage of good as well as from the bondage of evil. A golden chain is as much a chain as an iron one. Suppose there is a thorn in my finger. I use another to take the first one out, and when I have done so I throw both of them away; I have no need to keep the second thorn, because both are thorns after all. So the bad tendencies are to be counteracted by the good ones; the bad impressions in the mind should be removed by the waves of good impressions, until all that is evil almost disappears, or is subdued and held in control in a corner of the mind. But after that the good tendencies also have to be conquered. Thus the "attached" will become the "unattached." Work, but let not the action or the thought of it produce a deep impression on the mind. Let the ripples come and go; let huge actions proceed from the muscles and the brain, but let them not make any deep impression on the soul.

How can this be done? We see that the impression of any action to which we attach ourselves remains. I may meet hundreds of persons during the day, and among them see also one whom I love; and when I retire at night and try to think of all the faces I saw, the only face that comes before my mind is the face that I saw perhaps only for one minute and that I loved. All the others have vanished. My attachment to this particular person caused a very deep impression on my mind. Physiologically, the impressions have all been the same; every one of the different faces that I saw was pictured on the retina, and the brain took the picture in, and yet there was no similarity of effect upon the mind. Most of the faces, perhaps, were entirely new faces, about which I had never thought before; but that one face of which I got only a glimpse found associations inside. Perhaps I had pictured the person in my mind for years, knew hundreds of things about him, and this vision of him awakened hundreds of sleeping memories in my mind; this one impression, having been repeated perhaps a hundred times more than those of the different faces together, produced a great effect on the mind.

Therefore be unattached. Let things work; let the brain centres work; work incessantly, but let not a ripple conquer the mind. Work as if you were a stranger in this land, a sojourner. Work incessantly, but do not bind yourselves; bondage is terrible. This world is not our habitation, but only a stage through

which we are passing. Remember that great saying of
the Sāmkhya philosophy: "The whole of nature is for
the soul, not the soul for nature." The very reason
for nature's existence is the education of the soul;
it has no other meaning. It is there because the soul
must have knowledge, and through knowledge free
itself. If we remember this always, we shall never be
attached to nature; we shall know that nature is a
book which we are to read, and that when we have
gained the required knowledge the book is of no
more value to us. Instead of that, however, we
identify ourselves with nature; we think that the soul
is for nature, that the spirit is for the flesh, and, as
the common saying has it, we think that man "lives
to eat," not "eats to live." We are continually making
this mistake; we regard nature as the self and become
attached to it; and as soon as this attachment comes,
there is created in the soul a deep impression, which
binds us down and makes us work, not through freedom but like slaves.

The whole gist of this teaching is that you should
work as a master, not as a slave; work incessantly, but
do not do slave's work. Do you not see how everybody
works? Nobody can be altogether at rest. Ninety-nine
per cent of mankind work like slaves, and the result
is misery; it is all selfish work. Work through freedom! Work through love! The word *love* is very difficult to understand. Love never comes until there is
freedom. There is no true love possible in the slave.
If you buy a slave and tie him down in chains and
make him work for you, he will work like a drudge,
but there will be no love in him. So when we our-

selves work as slaves for the things of the world, there can be no love in us, and our work is not real work. This is true of work done for relatives and friends, and it is true of work done for our own selves. Selfish work is slave's work. And here is a test: Every act of love brings happiness; there is no act of love which does not bring peace and blessedness as its reaction. Real Existence, real Knowledge, and real Love are eternally connected with one another—the three in one. Where one of them is, the others also must be; they are the three aspects of the One without a second, Existence-Knowledge-Bliss. When that Existence becomes relative, we see it as the world; that Knowledge becomes in its turn modified into the knowledge of the things of the world; and that Bliss forms the foundation of all the love known to the heart of man. Therefore true love can never react so as to cause pain either to the lover or to the beloved. Suppose a man loves a woman. He wishes to have her all to himself and feels extremely jealous about her every movement; he wants her to sit near him, to stand near him, and to eat and move at his bidding. He is a slave to her and wishes to have her as his slave. That is not love; it is a kind of morbid affection of the slave, insinuating itself as love. It cannot be love, because it is painful; if she does not do what he wants, it brings him pain. With love there is no painful reaction; love brings only a reaction of bliss. If it does not, it is not love; it is a mistaking of something else for love. When you have succeeded in loving your husband, your wife, your children, the world, the whole universe, in such a manner that there is no reaction of pain or jealousy, no selfish feeling, then you are in a fit state to be unattached.

Krishna says: "Look at Me, Arjuna! If I stop working for one moment the whole universe will die. I have nothing to gain from work; I am the sole Lord. But why do I work? Because I love the world." God is unattached because He loves. That real love makes us unattached. Wherever there is attachment, the clinging to the things of the world, you must know that it is all physical attraction between particles of matter—something that attracts two bodies nearer and nearer all the time, and, if they cannot get near enough, produces pain. But where there is real love it does not rest on physical attraction at all. Such lovers may be a thousand miles away from one another, but their love will be there all the same; it does not die and will never produce any painful reaction.

To attain this non-attachment is almost a life-work; but as soon as we have reached this point we have attained the goal of love and become free. The bondage of nature falls away from us, and we see nature as it is; it forges no more chains for us. We stand entirely free and do not take the results of work into consideration. Who then cares what the results may be?

Do you ask anything of your children in return for what you have given them? It is your duty to work for them, and there the matter ends. In whatever you do for a particular person, city, or state, assume the same attitude towards it as you do towards your children—expect nothing in return. If you can invariably take the position of a giver, in which everything given by you is a free offering to the world, without any thought of return, then your work will bring you no attachment. Attachment comes only where we expect a return.

If working as slaves results in selfishness and attachment, working as masters of our own minds gives rise to the bliss of non-attachment. We often talk of right and justice, but we find that in the world right and justice are mere baby's talk. There are two things which guide the conduct of men: might and mercy. The exercise of might is invariably the exercise of selfishness. Men and women generally try to make the most of whatever power or advantage they have. Mercy is heaven itself; to be good we have all to be merciful. Even justice and right should stand on mercy. All thought of obtaining a return for the work we do hinders our spiritual progress; nay, in the end it brings misery.

There is another way in which this idea of mercy and selfless charity can be put into practice; that is by looking upon work as worship, if we believe in a Personal God. Here we give up all the fruits of our work unto the Lord; and worshipping Him thus, we have no right to expect anything from mankind for the work we do. The Lord Himself works incessantly and is ever without attachment. Just as water cannot wet the lotus leaf, so work cannot bind the unselfish man by giving rise to attachment to results. The selfless and unattached man may live in the very heart of a crowded and sinful city; he will not be touched by sin.

This idea of complete self-sacrifice is illustrated by the following story:

After the battle of Kurukshetra the five Pāndava brothers performed a great sacrifice and made very large gifts to the poor. All the people expressed amazement at the greatness and splendour of the sacrifice and said that such a sacrifice the world had never seen before. But after the ceremony there came a little mongoose; half his body was golden and the other half was brown; and he began to roll on the floor of the sacrificial hall. He said to those present: "You are all mistaken. This was no sacrifice." "What!" they exclaimed. "You say this was no sacrifice! Do you not know how money and jewels were poured out to the poor and everyone became rich and happy? This was the most wonderful sacrifice any man ever performed."

But the mongoose said: "There was once a little village, and in it there dwelt a poor brāhmin with his wife, his son, and his son's wife. They were very poor and lived on small gifts made to them for preaching and teaching. There came in that land a three years' famine, and the poor brāhmin suffered more than ever. At last, when the family had starved for days, the father brought home one morning a little barley flour, which he had been fortunate enough to obtain, and he divided it into four parts, one for each member of the family. They prepared it for their meal, and just as they were about to eat there was a knock at the door. The father opened it, and there stood a guest." (Now, in India a guest is a sacred person; he is like a god for the time being and must be treated as such.) "So the brāhmin said, 'Come in, sir; you are welcome.' He set before the guest his own portion of food. After quickly eating it the guest said: 'Oh, sir, you have almost killed me! I have been starving for ten days, and this little bit has but increased my hunger.' Then the wife said to her husband, 'Give him my share.' But the husband said, 'Not so.' The wife however insisted, saying: 'Here is a poor man. It is our duty as householders to see that he is fed, and it is my duty as a wife to give him my portion, seeing that you have no more to offer him.' Then she gave her share to the guest, after eating which he said he was still burning with hunger. So the son said: 'Take my portion also. It is the duty of a son to help his father to fulfil his obligations.' The guest ate that, but remained still unsatisfied; so the son's wife gave him her portion also. That was sufficient, and the guest departed, blessing them. That night those four people died of starvation. A few grains of that flour had fallen on the floor, and when I rolled my body on them half of it became golden, as you see. Since then I have been travelling all over the world, hoping to find another sacrifice like that. But nowhere have I found one; not even here has the other half of my body been turned into gold. That is why I say this was no sacrifice."

This idea of charity is going out of India; great men are becoming fewer and fewer. When I was first learning English I read an English story-book in which there was a story about a dutiful boy who had gone out to work and given some of his money to his old mother, and this act was praised for three or four pages. I was puzzled. No Hindu boy can ever understand the moral of that story. Now I understand it when I hear the Western idea, "every man for himself." And some men take everything for themselves, and fathers and mothers and wives and children go to the wall. That should never and nowhere be the ideal of the householder.

Now you see what karma-yoga means: even at the point of death to help anyone, without asking questions. Be cheated millions of times and never ask a question, and never think that you are doing good. Never vaunt of your gifts to the poor or expect their gratitude, but rather be grateful to them for giving you the occasion of practising charity towards them. Thus it is plain that to be an ideal householder is a much more difficult task than to be an ideal sannyāsin; the true life of action is indeed as hard as, if not harder than, the true life of renunciation.

WHAT IS DUTY?

IT IS NECESSARY in the study of karma-yoga to know what duty is. If I have to do something, I must first know that it is my duty, and then I can do it. The idea of duty, again, is different in different nations. The Mohammedan says that what is written in his book, the Koran, is his duty; the Hindu says that what is in the Vedas is his duty; and the Christian says that what is in the Bible is his duty. We find that there are varied ideas of duty, differing according to different states in life, different historical periods, and different nations.

The term *duty*, like every other universal, abstract term, is impossible to define clearly; we can only get an idea of it by knowing its practical operations and results. When certain things occur before us, we feel a natural or trained impulse to act in a certain manner towards them; when this impulse comes, the mind begins to think about the situation; sometimes it thinks that it is good to act in a particular manner under the given conditions, at other times it thinks that it is wrong to act in the same manner even in the very same circumstances. The ordinary idea of duty everywhere is that every good man follows the dictates of his conscience. But what is it that makes an act a duty? If a Christian finds a piece of beef before him and does not eat it to save his own life, or will not give it to save the life of another man, he is sure to feel that he has not done his duty. But if a

Hindu dares to eat that piece of beef or to give it to another Hindu, he is equally sure to feel that he too has not done his duty; the Hindu's training and education make him feel that way. In the last century there was a notorious band of robbers in India called Thugs. They thought it their duty to kill any man they could and take away his money; the larger the number of men they killed, the better they thought they were. Ordinarily, if a man goes out into the street and shoots down another man, he is apt to feel sorry for it, thinking that he has done wrong. But if the very same man, as a soldier in his regiment, kills not one but twenty, he is certain to feel glad and think that he has done his duty remarkably well.

Therefore we see that it is not the thing done that defines a duty. To give an objective definition of duty is thus impossible. Yet one can define duty from the subjective side. Any action that makes us go Godward is a good action and is our duty; any action that makes us go downward is evil and is not our duty. From the subjective standpoint we may see that certain acts have a tendency to exalt and ennoble us, while certain other acts have a tendency to degrade and brutalize us. But it is not possible to make out with certainty which acts have which kind of tendency in relation to all persons, of all sorts and conditions. There is, however, only one idea of duty which has been universally accepted by all mankind, of all ages and sects and countries, and it has been summed up in a Sanskrit aphorism thus: "Not injuring any living being is virtue; injuring any being is sin."

The Bhagavad Gītā frequently alludes to duties as

dependent upon birth and position in life. Birth and also position in life and society largely determine the mental and moral attitude of individuals towards the various activities of life. It is therefore our duty to do that work which will exalt and ennoble us in accordance with the ideals and activities of the society in which we are born. But it must be particularly remembered that the same ideals and activities do not prevail in all societies and countries; our ignorance of this is the main cause of much of the hatred of one nation towards another. An American thinks that whatever an American does in accordance with the customs of his country is the best thing to do, and that whoever does not follow his customs must be a very wicked man. A Hindu thinks that his customs are the only right ones and are the best in the world, and that whoever does not obey them must be the most wicked man living. This is quite a natural mistake, which all of us are apt to make. But it is very harmful; it is the cause of half the uncharitableness found in the world.

When I came to this country[1] and was going through the Chicago Fair, a man from behind pulled at my turban. I looked back and saw that he was a very gentlemanly-looking man, neatly dressed. I spoke to him and when he found that I knew English he became very much abashed. On another occasion in the same Fair a man gave me a push. When I asked him the reason, he also was ashamed and stammered out an apology saying, "Why do you dress that way?" The sympathies of these men were limited within the

[1] The United States of America.

range of their own language and their own fashion of dress. Much of the dislike felt by powerful nations for weaker ones is caused by this kind of prejudice, which dries up their fellow-feeling for others. That very man who asked me in Chicago why I did not dress as he did and wanted to ill-treat me because of my dress may have been a very good man, a good father and a good citizen; but the kindliness of his nature died out as soon as he saw a man in different dress. Foreigners are exploited in all countries, because they do not know how to defend themselves; thus they carry home false impressions of the peoples they have seen. Sailors, soldiers, and traders behave in foreign lands in very queer ways, although they would not dream of doing so in their own country; perhaps this is why the Chinese call Europeans and Americans "foreign devils." They would not do this if they saw the good, the kindly side of Western life.

Therefore the one point we ought to remember is that we should always try to see the duty of others through their own eyes and never judge the customs of other peoples by our own standard. I am not the standard of the universe. I have to accommodate myself to the world; the world does not have to adjust itself to me. So we see that environments change the nature of our duties, and doing the duty which is ours at any particular time is the best thing we can do in this world. Let us do the duty which is ours by birth; and when we have done that, let us do the duty which is ours by our position in life and in society. There is, however, one great danger in human nature —that is, that man never examines himself. He thinks he is quite as fit to be on the throne as the king. Even if he is, he must first show that he has done his duty in his own position; and then higher duties will come to him. When we begin to work earnestly in the world, nature gives us blows right and left and soon enables us to find out our position. No man can long occupy satisfactorily a position for which he is not fit. There is no use in grumbling against nature's adjustment. He who does the lower work is not therefore a lower man. No man is to be judged by the mere nature of his duties, but all should be judged by the manner and the spirit in which they perform them.

Later on we shall find that even this idea of duty undergoes change, and that the greatest work is done only when there is no selfish motive to prompt it. Yet it is work through the sense of duty that leads us to work without any idea of duty. Then work becomes worship—nay, something higher; then work is done for its own sake. We shall find that the goal of duty, either from the standpoint of ethics or of love, is the same as in all the other yogas, namely, to attenuate the lower self so that the Higher Self may shine forth, and to lessen the frittering away of energies on the lower plane of existence so that the soul may manifest them on the higher planes. This is accomplished by the constant denial of low desires, which duty rigorously requires. The whole organization of society has thus been developed consciously or unconsciously by means of action and experience. By limiting selfishness, we open the way to an unlimited expansion of the real nature of man.

Duty is seldom sweet. It is only when love greases

its wheels that it runs smoothly; otherwise it is a continuous friction. How else could parents do their duties to their children, husbands to their wives, and vice versa? Do we not meet with cases of friction every day in our lives? Duty is sweet only through love, and love shines alone in freedom. Yet is it freedom to be a slave to the senses, to anger, to jealousies, and to a hundred other petty things that occur every day in human life? In all these little roughnesses that we meet with in life the highest expression of freedom is to forbear. Women who are slaves to their own irritable, jealous tempers are apt to blame their husbands and assert their own "freedom"—as they think—not knowing that thereby they only prove that they are slaves. So it is with husbands who eternally find fault with their wives.

Chastity is the first virtue in man or woman, and the man who, however he may have strayed away, cannot be brought to the right path by a gentle and loving and chaste wife is indeed very rare. The world is not yet as bad as that. We hear much about brutal husbands all over the world and about the impurity of men, but is it not true that there are quite as many brutal and impure women as men? If all women were as good and pure as their own constant assertions would lead one to believe, I am perfectly satisfied that there would not be one impure man in the world. What brutality is there which purity and chastity cannot conquer? A good, chaste wife, who thinks of all men except her own husband as her children and has the attitude of a mother towards them, can grow so great in the power of her purity that there will not be a single man, however brutal, who will not breathe an atmosphere of holiness in her presence. Similarly, every husband must look upon all women, except his own wife, as he looks on his own mother or daughter or sister. That man, again, who wants to be a teacher of religion must look upon every woman as his mother and always behave towards her as such.

The position of the mother is the highest in the world, for it is the one place in which to learn and exercise the greatest unselfishness. The love of God is the only love that is higher than a mother's love; all other forms of love are lower. It is the duty of the mother to think of her children first and then of herself. But instead of that, if the parents are always thinking of themselves first, the result is that the relation between parents and children becomes the same as that between birds and their offspring; as soon as the latter are fledged, they do not recognize their parents. Blessed, indeed, is the man who can look upon woman as the representative of the Mother-hood of God. Blessed, indeed, is the woman to whom man represents the Fatherhood of God. Blessed are the children who look upon their parents as Divinity manifested on earth.

The only way to grow is to do the duty near at hand, and thus go on gathering strength till the highest state is reached. A young sannyāsin went to a forest. There he meditated, worshipped, and prac-tised yoga for a long time. After much hard work and practice, he was one day sitting under a tree, when some dry leaves fell upon his head. He looked up and saw a crow and a crane fighting on the top of

the tree, which made him very angry. He said,
"What! How dare you throw these dry leaves upon
my head?" As with these words he angrily looked
at them, a flash of fire went out—such was the yogi's
power—and burnt the birds to ashes. He was very
glad, almost overjoyed, at this development of power:
he could burn the crow and the crane by a look!
After a time he had to go to the town to beg his
bread. He stood at a door and called out, "Mother,
give me food." A voice came from inside the house:
"Wait a little, my son." The young man thought:
"You wretched woman, how dare you make me wait?
You do not yet know my power." While he was
thinking thus the voice said again: "Boy, don't be
thinking too much of yourself. Here is neither crow
nor crane." He was astonished. Still he had to wait.
At last the woman came, and he humbly said to her,
"Mother, how did you know that?" She said: "My
boy, I do not know your yoga or your other practices.
I am a simple, ordinary woman. I made you wait because my husband is ill and I was nursing him. All
my life I have struggled to do my duty. When I was
unmarried, I did my duty to my parents; now that I
am married, I do my duty to my husband. That is
all the yoga I practise. But by doing my duty I have
become illumined; thus I could read your thoughts
and know what you had done in the forest." She
further told him that if he wanted to know something
higher, he should go to the market of a certain town,
where he would find a *vyādha*[2] who would tell him

[2] One belonging to the lowest class of people, who were
hunters and butchers.

something that he would be very glad to learn. The sannyāsin thought, "Why should I go to that town, and to a vyādha?" But after what he had seen, his mind had opened a little; so he went. When he came to the town he found the market, and there saw, at a distance, a big fat vyādha cutting meat with a big knife, talking and bargaining with different people. The young man said: "Lord help me! Is this the man from whom I am going to learn? He is the incarnation of a demon, if he is anything." In the meantime the man looked up and said: "O Swami, did a lady send you here? Take a seat until I have done my business." The sannyāsin thought, "What comes to me here?" He took a seat, however. The man went on with his work, and after he had finished he took his money and said to the sannyāsin, "Come, sir; come to my home." On reaching home the vyādha gave him a seat, saying, "Wait here," and went into the house. He then bathed his old father and mother, fed them, and did all he could to please them, after which he came to the sannyāsin and said: "Now, sir, you have come here to see me. What can I do for you?" The sannyāsin asked him a few questions about the soul and about God, and the vyādha gave him a lecture which forms a part of the *Mahābhārata* called the *Vyādha Gītā*. It contains one of the highest flights of Vedānta. When the vyādha finished his teaching the sannyāsin felt astonished. He said: "Why are you in that body? With such knowledge as yours, why are you in a vyādha's body, and doing such filthy, ugly work?" "My son," replied the vyādha, "no duty is ugly, no duty is impure. My birth placed me in

these circumstances and this environment. In my boy-
hood I learnt the trade. I am unattached and I try
to do my duty well as a householder; I do all I can
to make my father and mother happy. I neither know
your yoga, nor have become a sannyāsin, nor have I
gone out of the world into a forest; nevertheless all
that I know has come to me through the unattached
doing of the duty which belongs to my position."

There is a sage in India, a great yogi, one of the
most wonderful men I have ever seen in my life.[3] He
is a peculiar man; he will not teach anyone. If you ask
him a question he will not answer. He hesitates to
take up the position of a teacher; he will not do it. If
you ask a question and wait for some days, in the
course of conversation he will bring up the subject,
and wonderful light will he throw on it. He told me
once the secret of work: "Let the end and the means
be one." When you are doing any work, do not think
of anything beyond. Do it as worship, as the highest
worship, and devote your whole life to it for the time
being. The vyādha and the woman in the story did
their duty with cheerfulness and whole-heartedness;
and the result was that they became illumined, thus
clearly showing that the right performance of the
duties of any station in life, without attachment to
results, leads us to the realization of the perfection of
the soul.

It is the worker attached to results who grumbles

[3] A reference to Pavhari Baba, whom Swami Vivekananda knew well. The Swami's meeting with the saint
is described on page 42 of *Vivekananda: A Biography*,
Ramakrishna-Vivekananda Center, New York, 1953.

about the nature of the duty which has fallen to his lot; to the unattached worker all duties are equally good and form efficient instruments with which selfishness and sensuality may be killed and the freedom of the soul secured. We are all apt to think too highly of ourselves. Our duties are determined by our deserts to a much larger extent than we are willing to grant. Competition rouses envy, and it kills the kindliness of the heart. To the grumbler all duties are distasteful; nothing will ever satisfy him, and his whole life is doomed to failure. Let us work on, doing whatever happens to be our duty, and be ever ready to put our shoulders to the wheel. Then surely we shall see the Light.

WE HELP OURSELVES, NOT
THE WORLD

B EFORE CONSIDERING further how devotion to duty
helps us in our spiritual progress, let me place
before you in brief another aspect of what we in India
mean by karma. In every religion there are three
parts: philosophy, mythology, and ritual. Philosophy,
of course, is the essence of every religion; mythology
explains and illustrates it by means of the more or less
legendary lives of great men, stories and fables of
wonderful things, and so on; ritual gives to that philosophy a still more concrete form, so that everyone
may grasp it—ritual is in fact concretized philosophy.
This ritual is karma. It is necessary in every religion,
because most of us cannot understand abstract spiritual things until we grow a great deal spiritually.

It is easy for men to think that they can understand everything, but when it comes to actual experience they find that abstract ideas are often very hard
to comprehend. Therefore symbols are of great help
and we cannot dispense with the symbolical method
of understanding abstract philosophical ideas. From
time immemorial all kinds of symbols have been used
by religions. In one sense we cannot think except in
symbols; words themselves are symbols of thought. In
another sense everything in the universe may be
looked upon as a symbol; the whole universe is a
symbol and God is the essence behind. This kind of
symbology is not simply the creation of man. Certain

people belonging to a religion did not sit down together and think out certain symbols, and bring them
into existence out of their own minds. The symbols
of religion have a natural growth. Otherwise, why is
it that certain symbols are associated with certain
ideas in the minds of almost everyone?

Certain symbols are universally prevalent. Many of
you may think that the cross first came into existence as
a symbol in connexion with the Christian religion;
but as a matter of fact it existed before Christianity,
before Moses was born, before the Vedas were revealed, even before there was any record of human
things. There is evidence that the cross was used by
the Aztecs and the Phoenicians; every race seems to
have had the cross. Again, the symbol of the crucified
Saviour, of a man crucified upon a cross, appears to
have been known to almost every nation. The circle
has been a great symbol throughout the world. Then
there is the most universal of all symbols, the swas-
tika. At one time it was thought that the Buddhists
carried it all over the world with them; but it has
been found out that ages before Buddhism it was
used by various nations. In Babylon and in Egypt it
was also in use. What does this show? It shows that
all these symbols could not have been purely conven-
tional. There must be some reason for their use, some
natural association between them and the human
mind.

Language is not the result of convention; it is not a
fact that people ever agreed to represent certain ideas
by certain words. There never was an idea without
a corresponding word or a word without a correspond-

ing idea. Ideas and words are in their nature inseparable. The symbols to represent ideas may be sound-symbols or colour-symbols. Deaf-and-dumb people have to think with other than sound-symbols. Every thought in the mind has a form as its counterpart; this is called in Sanskrit philosophy nāma-rupa—"name and form." It is as impossible to create by convention a system of symbols as it is to create a language.

In the world's ritualistic symbols we have an expression of the religious thought of humanity. It is easy to say that there is no use for rituals and temples and all such paraphernalia; every baby says that in modern times. But it must be easy for all to see that those who worship inside a temple are in many respects different from those who will not worship there. Therefore the association of particular temples, rituals, and other concrete forms with particular religions has a tendency to bring into the minds of the followers of those religions the thoughts for which those concrete things stand as symbols; and it is not wise to ignore rituals and symbology altogether. The study and practice of these things naturally form a part of karma-yoga.

There are many other aspects of this science of work. One among them is to know the relation between thought and word, and what can be achieved by the power of the word. In every religion the power of the word is recognized—so much so that in some of them creation itself is said to have come out of the Word. The external aspect of the thought of God is the Word, and because God thought and willed before He created, creation came out of the Word.

In this stress and hurry of our materialistic life our nerves lose sensitivity and become hardened. The older we grow and the longer we are knocked about in the world, the more callous we become; and we are apt to neglect even things that happen persistently and prominently around us. Human nature, however, asserts itself sometimes and we are led to inquire into and wonder at some of these common occurrences. Wondering is thus the first step in the acquisition of wisdom. Apart from the higher philosophic and religious value of the Word, we can see that sound-symbols play a prominent part in the drama of human life. I am talking to you. The vibrations of the air caused by my speaking go into your ears; they touch your nerves and produce effects in your minds. You cannot resist this. What could be more wonderful than this? One man calls another a fool, and this other stands up and clenches his fist and lands a blow on his nose. Look at the power of words! There is a woman weeping and miserable; another woman comes along and speaks a few gentle words to her; the doubled-up frame of the weeping woman becomes straight at once; her sorrow is gone and soon she begins to smile. Think of the power of the words! They are as great a force in common life as they are in higher philosophy. Day and night we manipulate this force without thought and without inquiry. To know the nature of this force and to use it well is also a part of karma-yoga.

Our duty to others means helping others, doing good to the world. Why should we do good to the world? Apparently to help the world, but really to

help ourselves. We should always try to help the
world. That should be the highest motive in us. But
if we consider well, we find that the world does not
require our help at all. This world was not made that
you or I should come and help it. I once read a
sermon in which it was said: "All this beautiful world
is very good, because it gives us time and opportunity
to help others." Apparently this is a very beautiful
sentiment; but is it not blasphemy to say that the
world needs our help? We cannot deny that there is
much misery in it; to go out and help others is, therefore, the best thing we can do, although, in the long
run, we shall find that by helping others we only
help ourselves. As a boy I had some white mice.
They were kept in a little box in which there were
little wheels, and when the mice tried to cross the
wheels, the wheels turned and turned, and the mice
never got anywhere. So it is with the world and our
helping it. The only gain is that we get moral exercise.

This world is neither good nor evil; each man manu-
factures a world for himself. If a blind man thinks
of the world, he will think of it as soft or hard, cold
or hot. We are a mass of happiness or misery; we
have seen that hundreds of times in our lives. As a
rule the young are optimistic and the old pessimistic.
The young have life before them; the old complain
that their day is gone; hundreds of desires, which they
cannot fulfil, struggle in their hearts. Both are foolish
nevertheless. Life is good or evil according to the state
of mind in which we look at it; it is neither in itself.
Fire, in itself, is neither good nor evil. When it keeps

us warm we say, "How beautiful fire is!" When it burns our fingers we curse it. Still, in itself it is neither good nor bad; according as we use it, it produces in us the feeling of good or bad. So also is this world. It is perfect. By perfection I mean that it is perfectly fitted to meet its ends. We may all be perfectly sure that it will go on beautifully without us, and we need not bother our heads with wishing to help it.

Yet we must do good; the desire to do good is the highest motive power we have. But we must remember that it is a privilege to help others. Do not stand on a high pedestal and take five cents in your hand and say, "Here, my poor man!" But be grateful that the poor man is there, so that by making a gift to him you are able to help yourself. It is not the receiver that is blessed, but it is the giver. Be thankful that you are allowed to exercise your power of benevolence and mercy in the world, and thus become pure and perfect. All good acts tend to make us pure and perfect. What can we do at best? Build a hospital, make roads, or erect charity asylums! We may organize a charity and collect two or three millions of dollars, build a hospital with one million, with the second give balls and drink champagne, and of the third let the officers steal half, and leave the rest finally to reach the poor—but what are all these? One mighty wind in five minutes can break all your buildings up. What shall we do then? One volcanic eruption may sweep away all our roads and hospitals and cities and buildings. Let us give up all this foolish talk of doing good to the world. It is not waiting for

your or my help. Yet we must work and constantly
do good, because it is a blessing to ourselves. That
is the only way we can become perfect. No beggar
whom we have helped has ever owed a single cent to
us; we owe everything to him, because he has allowed us to exercise our charity on him. It is entirely wrong to think that we have done, or can do,
good to the world, or to think that we have helped
certain people. It is a foolish thought, and all foolish
thoughts bring misery. We think that we have helped
some man and expect him to thank us; and because
he does not, unhappiness comes to us. Why should
we expect anything in return for what we do? Be
grateful to the man you help. Think of him as God.
Is it not a great privilege to be allowed to worship
God by helping our fellow man? If we were really
unattached, we should escape all this pain of vain
expectation and could cheerfully do good work in
the world. Never will unhappiness or misery come
through work done without attachment. The world
will go on with its happiness and misery through
eternity.

There was a poor man who wanted some money,
and someone had told him that if he could get hold
of a ghost, he might command him to bring money
or anything else he liked; so he was very anxious to
get hold of a ghost. He went about searching for a
man who would give him a ghost; and at last he
found a sage with yogic powers, and besought his
help. The sage asked him what he would do with a
ghost. "I want a ghost to work for me. Teach me
how to get hold of one, sir; I desire it very much,"

replied the man. But the sage said, "Don't disturb yourself; go home." The next day the man went again to the sage and began to weep and pray, "Give me a ghost; I must have a ghost, sir, to help me." At last the sage was disgusted and said: "Here is a magic word for you. Repeat it and a ghost will come; and whatever you say to him he will do. But beware; these ghosts are terrible beings and must be kept continually busy. If you fail to give them work they will take your life." The man replied, "That is easy; I can give him enough work for his whole life." Then he went to a forest and repeated the magic word for a long while, when a huge ghost appeared before him and said: "I am a ghost. I have been conquered by your magic; but you must keep me constantly employed. The moment you fail to give me work I will kill you." The man said, "Build me a palace," and the ghost said, "It is done; the palace is built." "Bring me money," said the man. "Here is your money," said the ghost. "Cut this forest down and build a city in its place." "That is done," said the ghost; "anything more?" Now the man began to be frightened and thought, "I can give him nothing more to do; he does everything in a trice." The ghost said, "Give me something to do or I will eat you up." The poor man could find no further occupation for him and was frightened. So he ran and ran and at last reached the sage, and said, "Oh, sir, save my life!" The sage asked him what the matter was, and the man replied: "I have nothing to give the ghost to do. Everything I tell him to do he does in a moment, and he threatens to eat me up if I do not give him work." Just then the ghost arrived, saying, "I'll eat you up," and he was about to swallow the man. The man began to tremble, and begged the sage to save his life. The sage said: "I will find you a way out. Do you see that dog with a, curly tail? Draw your sword quickly and cut his tail off and give it to the ghost to straighten out." The man cut off the dog's tail and gave it to the ghost, saying, "Straighten that out for me." The ghost took it and slowly and carefully straightened it out, but as soon as he let it go, it instantly curled up again. Once more he laboriously straightened it out, only to find that again it curled up as soon as he let it go. Once more he patiently straightened it out, but as soon as he let it go it curled up again. So he went on for days and days, until he was exhausted and said: "I was never in such trouble before in my life. I am an old, veteran ghost, but never before was I in such trouble. I will make a compromise with you. You let me off and I will let you keep all I have given you and will promise not to harm you." The man was much pleased and accepted the offer gladly.

This world is like a dog's curly tail, and people have been striving to straighten it out for hundreds of years; but when they let it go, it curls up again. How could it be otherwise? When we know that this world is like a dog's curly tail and will never be straightened, we shall not become fanatics. One must first know how to work without attachment; then one will not be a fanatic. If there were no fanaticism in the world it would make much more progress than it does now. It is a mistake to think that fanaticism can make for the progress of mankind. On the contrary, it is a retarding element, creating hatred and anger, causing people to fight each other, and making them unsympathetic. We think that whatever we do or possess is the best in the world, and what we do not do or possess is of no value. So always remember the instance of the dog's curly tail whenever you have a tendency to become a fanatic. You need not worry or make yourself sleepless about the world; it will go on without you. When you have avoided fanaticism, then alone will you work well. It is the level-headed man, the calm man of good judgement and cool nerves, of great sympathy and love, who does good work and so does good to himself. The fanatic is foolish and has no sympathy; he can never straighten out the world, nor can he himself become pure and perfect.

To recapitulate the chief points in today's lecture: First, we have to bear in mind that we are all debtors to the world and that the world does not owe us anything. It is a great privilege for all of us to be allowed to do anything for the world. In helping the world we really help ourselves. The second point is that there is a God in this universe. It is not true that this universe is drifting and stands in need of help from you and me. God is ever present therein; He is undying and eternally active and infinitely watchful. When the whole universe sleeps He sleeps not; He is working incessantly; all the changes in the world are caused by Him. Thirdly, we ought not to hate anyone. This world will always continue to be a mixture of good and evil. Our duty is to sympathize with the weak and to love even the wrongdoer. The world is a grand moral gymnasium wherein we all have to take exercise so that we shall become stronger and stronger spiritually. Fourthly, we ought not to be fanatics of any kind, because fanaticism is opposed to love. You hear fanatics glibly saying, "I do not hate the sinner; I hate the sin"; but I am prepared to go any distance to see the face of that man who can really make a distinction between the sin and the sinner. It is easy to say so. If we can distinguish well between quality and substance we may become perfect men. It is not easy to do this. And further, the calmer we are and the less disturbed our nerves, the more shall we love and the better will our work be.

NON-ATTACHMENT IS COMPLETE
SELF-ABNEGATION

JUST AS EVERY ACTION that emanates from us comes back to us as reaction, even so our actions may act on other people and theirs on us. Perhaps all of you have observed that when persons do evil work they become more and more evil, and that when they begin to do good they become better and better and learn to do good at all times. This intensification of the influence of action cannot be explained on any other ground than that we act and react upon each other. When I am doing a certain work, my mind may be said to be in a certain state of vibration; all minds which are in a similar state will have the tendency to be affected by my mind. To take an illustration from physical science: Suppose there are different musical instruments tuned alike in one room; you may have noticed that when one is struck the others have a tendency to vibrate so as to give the same note. So all minds that have the same tension, so to say, will be equally affected by the same thought. Of course, this influence of thought on mind will vary, according to distance and other causes, but the mind is always open to being affected. Suppose I am doing an evil act; my mind is in a certain state of vibration, and all minds in the universe which are in a similar state have a tendency to be affected by the vibration of my mind. So, when I am doing a good action, my mind is in another state

of vibration, and all minds similarly strung have a
tendency to be affected by my mind; and this power
of mind upon mind is greater or less according as the
force of the tension is greater or less.

Following this simile further, it is quite possible
that, just as light-waves may travel for millions of
years before they reach any object, so thought-waves
too may travel hundreds of years before they meet an
object with which they will vibrate in unison. It is
quite possible, therefore, that this atmosphere of ours
is full of such thought-vibrations, both good and evil.
Every thought projected from every brain goes on vi-
brating, as it were, until it meets an object fit to receive it. Any mind which is capable of receiving some
of these impulses will take them immediately. So
when a man is doing evil actions he has brought his
mind to a certain state of tension, and all the waves
corresponding to that state of tension, which may be
said to be already in the atmosphere, will struggle
to enter into his mind. That is why an evil-doer generally goes on doing more and more evil. His actions
become intensified. Such, also, is true of the doer of
good; he will open himself to all the good waves that
are in the atmosphere, and his good actions also will
become intensified. We run, therefore, a two-fold
danger in doing evil: first, we open ourselves to all
the evil influence surrounding us; secondly, we create
evil which will affect others perhaps hundreds of years
hence. In doing evil we injure ourselves and others
also. In doing good we do good to ourselves and to
others as well; and like all other forces in man, these

forces of good and evil also gather strength from outside.

According to karma-yoga, the action one has done cannot be destroyed until it has borne fruit; no power in nature can stop it from yielding its results. If I do an evil deed I must suffer for it; there is no power in this universe to stop or stay it. Similarly, if I do a good deed there is no power in the universe which can stop its bearing good results. The cause must have its effect; nothing can prevent or restrain this.

Now comes a very fine and serious point in karma-yoga, namely, that these actions of ours, both good and evil, are intimately connected with each other. We cannot draw a line of demarcation and say that one action is entirely good and another entirely evil. There is no action which does not bear good and evil fruits at the same time. To take the nearest example: I am talking to you, and some of you, perhaps, think I am doing good; and at the same time I am surely killing thousands of microbes in the atmosphere. I am thus doing evil to something else. When an action affects, in a good manner, those whom we know and who are very dear to us, we say that it is a very good action. For instance, you may call my speaking to you very good, but the microbes will not; the microbes you do not see, but yourselves you do see. The way in which my talk affects you is obvious to you, but how it affects the microbes is not so obvious. And so, too, if we analyse our evil actions, we may find that some good possibly results from them somewhere. He who sees that in good action there is something evil, and that in evil action there is some good somewhere, has known the secret of work.

But what follows from this? That howsoever we may try, there cannot be any action which is perfectly pure or any which is perfectly impure, taking purity and impurity in the sense of injury and non-injury. We cannot breathe or live without injuring others, and every bit of the food we eat is taken away from another's mouth; our very lives are crowding out other lives. It may be men or animals or microbes, but some one or other of these we have to crowd out. That being the case, it naturally follows that perfection can never be attained by work. We may work through all eternity, but there will be no way out of this intricate maze. You may work on and on and on; there will be no end to this inevitable association of good and evil in the results of work.

The second point to consider is: What is the end of work? We find that the vast majority of people in every country believe that there will be a time when this world shall become perfect, when there shall be no disease or death or unhappiness or wickedness. That is a very good idea, a very good motive power to inspire and uplift the ignorant; but if we think for a moment, we shall find on the very face of it that it cannot be so. How can it be, seeing that good and evil are the obverse and reverse of the same coin? How can you have good without evil at the same time? What is meant by perfection? A perfect life is a contradiction in terms. Life itself is a state of continuous struggle between ourselves and everything outside. Every moment we are actually fighting with external nature, and if we are defeated our life must go. There is, for instance, a continual struggle for food and air. If food or air fails we die. Life is not a simple and smoothly flowing thing; it is a complex affair. This struggle between something inside and the external world is what we call life. So it is clear that when this struggle ceases there will be an end of life. What is meant by ideal happiness is this: the cessation of struggle. But then life too will cease, for the struggle can cease only when life itself has ceased.

We have seen already that in helping the world we help ourselves. The main effect of work done for others is that it purifies us. By means of the constant effort to do good to others we are attempting to forget ourselves; this forgetfulness of self is the one great lesson we have to learn in life. Man foolishly thinks that through selfish action he can make himself happy; but after years of struggle he finds out at last that true happiness consists in killing selfishness and that no one can make him happy except himself. Every act of charity, every thought of sympathy, every act of help, every good deed, takes so much of self-importance away from our little selves and makes us think of ourselves as the lowest and the least; and therefore they are all good. Here we find that jnāna, bhakti, and karma all come to one point. The highest idea is eternal and entire self-abnegation, where there is no "I," but all is "Thou"; and whether he is conscious or unconscious of it, karma-yoga leads man to that end. A religious preacher may become horrified at the idea of an Impersonal God; he may insist on a Personal God and wish to maintain his own identity and individuality, whatever he may mean by that. But his ideas of ethics, if they are really good, cannot but be based on the highest self-abnegation. This is the basis of all morality. You may extend it to men or animals or angels; it is the one basic idea, the one fundamental principle, running through all ethical systems.

You will find various classes of men in this world. First, there are the godly men, whose self-abnegation is complete and who do only good to others even at the sacrifice of their own lives. These are the highest of men. If there are a hundred of such in any country, that country need never despair. But they are unfortunately too few. Then there are the good men, who do good to others so long as it does not injure themselves. And there is a third class, who, to do good to themselves, injure others. It is said by a Sanskrit poet that there is a fourth unnameable class of people, who injure others merely for injury's sake. Just as there are at one pole of existence supremely good men, who do good for the sake of doing good, so, at the other pole, there are men who injure others just for the sake of the injury. They do not gain anything thereby, but it is their nature to do evil.

Here are two Sanskrit words. The one is *pravritti*, which means "revolving towards," and the other is *nivritti*, which means "revolving away from." The "revolving towards" is what we call the world: the "me" and "mine." It includes all those things which are always pampering that "me" by wealth and position and power and name and fame, and which are of a grasping nature, always tending to accumulate everything in one centre, that centre being "myself." That is pravritti, the natural tendency of every human being—taking everything from everywhere and heaping it around one centre, that centre being man's own sweet self. When this tendency begins to break and is replaced by nivritti, or "revolving away from," then begin morality and religion. Both pravritti and nivritti are of the nature of work: the former is evil work, and the latter is good work.

Nivritti is the fundamental basis of all morality and religion; and the very culmination of it is entire self-abnegation, readiness to sacrifice mind and body and everything for another being. When a man has reached that state he has attained to the perfection of karma-yoga. This is the highest result of good works. Although a man has not studied a single system of philosophy, although he does not believe in any God and never has believed, although he has not prayed even once in his whole life, if the simple power of good actions has brought him to that state where he is ready to give up his life and all else for others, he has arrived at the same point to which the religious man will come through his prayers and the philosopher through his knowledge. So you find that the philosopher, the worker, and the devotee all meet at one point, that one point being self-abnegation.

However much the various systems of philosophy and religion may differ, all mankind stands in reverence and awe before the man who is ready to sacrifice himself for others. Here it is not at all a question of creed or doctrine. Even men who are very much opposed to all religious ideas feel, when they see one of these acts of complete self-sacrifice, that they must revere it. And have you not seen even a most bigoted Christian, when he reads Edwin Arnold's *The Light of Asia,* stand in reverence of Buddha, who preached no God, preached nothing but self-sacrifice? The only thing is that the bigot does not know that his own end and aim in life is exactly the same as that of those with whom he differs.

The worshipper, by keeping constantly before him the idea of God and living in holy surroundings, comes to the same point at last and says, "Thy will be done"; he keeps nothing for himself. That is self-abnegation. The philosopher, with his knowledge, sees that the seeming self is a delusion and easily gives it up. That too is self-abnegation. So karma, bhakti, and jnāna all meet here; and this is what was meant by all the great preachers of ancient times when they taught that God is not the world. The world is one thing and God is another; and this distinction is very true. What they mean by the world is selfishness. Unselfishness is God. One man may be living on a throne, in a golden palace, and be perfectly unselfish; then he is in God. Another may live in a hut and wear rags and have nothing in the world; yet if he is selfish, he is an intensely worldly man.

To come back to one of our main points: We say that we cannot do good without at the same time doing some evil, or do evil without doing some good. Knowing this, how can we work? There have therefore been sects in this world which have in an astoundingly preposterous way preached slow suicide as the only means to get out of the world; because if a man lives he has to kill poor little animals and plants or do injury to something or someone. So, according to them, the only way out of the world is to die. The Jains have preached this doctrine as their highest ideal and it seems to be very logical. But the true solution is found in the Gitā. It is the doctrine of non-attachment—to be attached to nothing while doing our duty in life. Know that you are separated entirely from the world; that you are in the world but not of it, and that whatever you may be doing in it you are not doing for your own sake. Any action that you do for yourself will bring its effect to bear upon you. If it is a good action, you will have to take the good result, and if a bad action, you will have to take the bad result; but any action that is not done for your own sake, whatever it be, will not affect you. There is to be found a very expressive sentence in our scriptures, embodying this idea: Even if a man kills the whole universe or is himself killed, he is neither the killer nor the killed, when he knows that he is not acting for himself at all.

Therefore karma-yoga teaches: "Do not give up the world. Live in the world, imbibe its ideas as much as you can." But are these for your own enjoyment's sake? Certainly not. Enjoyment should not be the goal. First kill your self and then regard the whole world as yourself. "The old man must die," as the Christians used to say. This "old man" is the selfish idea that the whole world is made for our enjoyment. Foolish parents teach their children to pray, "O Lord, Thou hast created this sun for me and this moon for me"—as if the Lord had nothing else

to do than to create everything for these babies. Do
not teach your children such nonsense. Then again,
there are people who are foolish in another way:
They teach us that all these animals were created
for us to kill and eat, and that this universe is for
the enjoyment of men. That is all foolishness. A
tiger may say, "Man was created for me," and complain: "Lord, how wicked are these men, who do not
come and place themselves before me to be eaten!
They are breaking Your law." If the world is created
for us we are also created for the world. That this
world is created for our enjoyment is the most wicked
idea that holds us down. This world is not for our
sake. Millions pass out of it every year; the world does
not feel it; millions of others take their place. Just
as much as the world is created for us, so also are we
created for the world.

To work properly, therefore, you have first to give
up the idea of attachment. Secondly, do not mix in
the fray; hold yourself as a witness and go on working. My Master used to say, "Look upon your children as a nurse does." The nurse will love your baby
and fondle it and play with it and behave towards it
as gently as if it were her own child; but as soon as
you give her notice to quit, she is ready to start off
with bag and baggage from the house—everything in
the shape of attachment is forgotten. It will not give
the ordinary nurse the least pang to leave your children and take care of other children. Even so should
be your attitude towards all that you consider your
own. You are like the nurse; if you believe in God,

believe that all these things which you consider yours are really His.

The greatest weakness often insinuates itself as the greatest good and strength. It is a weakness to think that anyone is dependent on me and that I can do good to another. This belief is the mother of all our attachment, and through this attachment comes all our pain. We must inform our minds that no one in this universe depends upon us; not one beggar depends on our charity, not one soul on our kindness, not one living thing on our help. All are helped on by nature and would be so helped even though millions of us were not here. The course of nature will not stop for such as you and me; it is, as already pointed out, only a blessed privilege to you and to me that we are allowed, through helping others, to educate ourselves. This is a great lesson to learn in life, and when we have learnt it fully we shall never be unhappy; we can go and mix without harm in society anywhere and everywhere. You may have wives or husbands, and regiments of servants, and kingdoms to govern; but if you act on the principle that the world is not for you and does not inevitably need you, they can do you no harm. This very year some of your friends may have died. Has the world stopped moving? Is it waiting for their coming back? Is everything standing still? No, it is not. So drive out of your mind the idea that you have to do something for the world; the world does not require any help from you. It is sheer nonsense on the part of any man to think that he is born to help

the world. It is simply vanity; it is selfishness insinuating itself in the form of virtue.

When you have trained your mind and your nerves
to realize this idea of the world's non-dependence on
you or on anybody, there will then be no reaction in
the form of pain resulting from work. When you give
something to a man and expect nothing—do not even
expect the man to be grateful—his ingratitude will
not tell upon you, because you never expected anything, never thought you had any right to anything
in the way of a return. You gave him what he deserved; his own karma got it for him; your karma
made you the carrier of it. Why should you be proud
of having given away something? You were the bearer
who carried the money or other kind of gift, and
the man deserved it by his own karma. Where then
is the reason for pride in you? There is nothing very
great in what you give to the world. When you have
acquired the feeling of non-attachment, there will
then be neither good nor evil for you. It is only selfishness that causes the difference between good and evil.

It is a very hard thing to understand, but you will
come to learn in time that nothing in the universe
has power over you until you allow it to exercise
such power. Nothing has power over the Self of man
until the Self becomes a fool and loses independence.
So by non-attachment you overcome and deny the
power of anything to act upon you. It is very easy
to say that nothing has the right to act upon you until
you allow it to do so; but what is the true sign of
the man who really does not allow anything to work
upon him, who is neither happy nor unhappy when

acted upon by the external world? The sign is that
good or ill fortune causes no change in his mind; in
all conditions he remains the same.

There was a great sage in India named Vyāsa. This
Vyāsa is known as the author of the *Vedānta Sutras*
and was a holy man. His father had tried to become
a very perfect man and had failed. His grandfather
had also tried and failed. His great-grandfather had
likewise tried and failed. He himself did not succeed
fully, but his son, Śuka, was born perfect. Vyāsa
taught his son wisdom, and after teaching him the
knowledge of Truth himself, he sent him to the court
of King Janaka. Janaka was a great king and was
called Janaka Videha. Videha means "without a
body." Although a king, he had entirely forgotten
that he had a body; he felt all the time that he was
Spirit. The boy Śuka was sent to be taught by him.
The king knew that Vyāsa's son was coming to him
to learn wisdom; so he made certain arrangements
beforehand. When the boy presented himself at the
gate of the palace, the guards took no notice of him
whatsoever. They only gave him a seat, and he sat
there for three days and nights, nobody speaking to
him, nobody asking him who he was or whence he
came. He was the son of a very great sage; his father
was honoured by the whole country; and he himself
was a most respectable person; yet the low, vulgar
guards of the palace would take no notice of him.
Then, suddenly, the ministers of the king and all the
great officials came and received him with the greatest
honours. They conducted him in and showed him into
splendid rooms, gave him the most fragrant baths

and wonderful dress, and for eight days they kept him there in all kinds of luxury. The solemnly serene face of Śuka did not change even to the smallest extent by the change in the treatment accorded to him; he was the same in the midst of this luxury as when waiting at the door. Then he was brought before the king. The king was on his throne, music was playing, and dancing and other amusements were going on. The king gave him a cup of milk, full to the brim, and asked him to go seven times round the hall without spilling even a drop. The boy took the cup and proceeded in the midst of the music and the attraction of the beautiful faces. As the king had asked, seven times did he go round, and not a drop of the milk was spilt. The boy's mind could not be attracted by anything in the world unless he allowed it to affect him. And when he brought the cup to the king, the king said to him: "What your father has taught you, and what you have learnt yourself, I can only repeat. You have known the Truth. Go home."

Thus the man who has practised control over himself cannot be acted upon by anything outside; there is no more slavery for him; his mind has become free. Such a man alone has earned the right to live well in the world. We generally find men holding two opinions regarding the world. Some are pessimists and say: "How horrible this world is! How wicked!" Others are optimists and say: "How beautiful this world is! How wonderful!" To those who have not controlled their own minds, the world is either full of evil or at best a mixture of good and evil. This very world will become to us a happy world when we become masters of our own minds. Nothing will then work upon us as good or evil; we shall find everything to be in its proper place, to be harmonious. Often men who begin by saying that the world is a hell end by saying that it is a heaven, when they succeed in the practice of self-control. If we want to be karma-yogis and wish to train ourselves for the attainment of this state, wherever we may begin we are sure to end in perfect self-abnegation; and as soon as this seeming self has gone, the whole world, which at first appears to us to be filled with evil, will appear to be heaven itself and full of blessedness. Its very atmosphere will be blessed; every human face there will be good. Such is the end and aim of karma-yoga, and such is its perfection in practical life.

Our various yogas do not conflict with each other; each of them leads us to the same goal and makes us perfect; only each has to be strenuously practised. The whole secret is in practising. First you have to hear, then think, and then practise. This is true of every yoga. You have first to hear about it and understand what it is; and many things which you do not understand will be made clear to you by constant hearing and thinking. It is hard to understand everything at once. The explanation of everything is after all in yourself. No one is ever really taught by another; each of us has to teach himself. The external teacher offers only the suggestion, which arouses the internal teacher, who helps us to understand things. Then things will be made clearer to us by our own power of perception and thought, and we shall realize them in our own souls; and that realization will grow into intense power of will. First it is feeling, then it becomes willing, and out of that willing comes tremendous force for work, which will go through every vein and nerve and muscle, until the whole mass of the body is changed into an instrument of the yoga of unselfish work, and the desired result of perfect self-abnegation and utter unselfishness is duly attained. This attainment does not depend on any dogma or doctrine or belief. Whether one is Christian or Jew or Hindu, it does not matter. Are you unselfish? That is the question. If you are, you will be perfect without reading a single religious book, without going into a single church or temple. Each one of our yogas is fitted to make men perfect even without the help of the others, because they all have the same goal in view. The yogas of work, wisdom, and devotion are all capable of serving as direct and independent means for the attainment of moksha. "Fools alone say that work and philosophy are different, not the learned." The learned know that, though apparently different from each other, they at last lead to the same goal of human perfection.

FREEDOM

W<small>E HAVE STATED THAT</small> in addition to meaning work, psychologically the word *karma* also implies causation. Any word, any action, any thought, that produces an effect is called a karma. Thus the law of karma means the law of causation, of inevitable cause and sequence. Wheresoever there is a cause, there an effect must be produced; this necessity cannot be resisted; and this law of karma, according to our philosophy, is true throughout the whole universe. Whatever we see or feel or do, whatever action there is anywhere in the universe, while being on the one hand the effect of past work, becomes, on the other, a cause in its turn and produces its own effect.

It is necessary, together with this, to consider what is meant by the word *law*. By law is meant the tendency of a series to repeat itself. When we see one event followed by another, or sometimes happening simultaneously with another, we expect this sequence or coexistence to recur. Our old logicians and philosophers of the Nyāya school call this law by the name of vyāpti. According to them all our ideas of law are due to association. A series of phenomena becomes associated with certain things in our mind in a sort of invariable order; so whatever we perceive at any time is immediately referred to similar facts in the mind. Any one idea or, according to our psychology, any one wave that is produced in the

mind-stuff, or chitta, must always give rise to many
similar waves. This is the psychological idea of association, and causation is only an aspect of this grand
pervasive principle of association. This pervasiveness
of association is what is, in Sanskrit, called vyāpti.
In the external world the idea of law is the same as
in the internal—the expectation that a particular
phenomenon will be followed by another and that
the series will repeat itself. Strictly speaking, therefore, law does not exist in nature. It is really an error
to say that gravitation exists in the earth or that there
is any law existing objectively anywhere in nature.
Law is the method, the manner, in which our mind
grasps a series of phenomena; it is all in the mind.
Certain phenomena, happening one after another,
or together, and followed by the conviction of the
regularity of their recurrence, thus enabling our
minds to grasp the method of the whole series, are
explained by what we call law.

The next question for consideration is what we
mean by law's being universal. Our universe is that
portion of Existence which is conditioned by what
the Sanskrit philosophers call deśa-kāla-nimitta, or
what is known to European philosophy as space, time,
and causation. This universe is only a part of Infinite
Existence, thrown into a peculiar mould composed of
space, time, and causation. It necessarily follows that
law is possible only within this conditioned universe;
beyond it there cannot be any law. When we speak
of the universe we mean only that portion of Existence which is limited by our minds—the universe of
the senses, which we can see, feel, touch, hear, think

of, imagine. This alone is under law; but beyond it,
Existence cannot be subject to law, because causation
does not extend beyond the world of our minds. Anything beyond the range of the mind and the senses
is not bound by the law of causation, because there
is no mental association of things in the region beyond the senses, and no causation is possible without
association of ideas. It is only when Being or Existence becomes moulded into name and form that it
obeys the law of causation and is said to be subject
to law—because all law has its essence in causation.

Therefore we see at once that there cannot be any
such thing as free will; the very words are a contradiction, because the will is something that we know,
and everything that we know is within our universe,
and everything within our universe is moulded by
the conditions of space, time, and causation. Everything that we know, or can possibly know, must be
subject to causation, and that which obeys the law
of causation cannot be free. It is acted upon by other
agents and becomes a cause in its turn. But that
which has become converted into the will, which
was not the will before, but which, when it fell into
this mould of space, time, and causation, became
converted into the human will, is free; and when this
will gets out of the mould of space, time, and causation, it will be free again. From freedom it comes,
and it falls into the mould of bondage, and it gets out
and goes back to freedom again.

The question has been raised as to whence this
universe comes, in what it rests, and whither it goes;
and the answer has been given that from freedom

it comes, in bondage it rests, and into that freedom it goes back again. So when we speak of man as no other than the Infinite Being, which is manifesting Itself through him, we mean that only one very small part thereof is man; this body and this mind which we see are only one part of the whole, only one speck in the Infinite Being. This whole universe is only one speck in the Infinite Being; and all our laws, our bondages, our joys and our sorrows, our happinesses and our expectations, are only within this small universe; all our progression and regression are within its small compass. So you see how childish it is to expect a continuation of this universe—the creation of our minds—and to expect to go to heaven, which after all must mean only a repetition of this world that we know. You see at once that it is an impossible and childish desire to make the whole of Infinite Existence conform to the limited and conditioned existence which we know. When a man says that he will have again and again this same thing which he is having now, or, as I sometimes put it, when he asks for a *comfortable* religion, you may know that he has become so degenerate that he cannot think of anything higher than what he is now, anything beyond his insignificant present surroundings. He has forgotten his infinite nature, and his whole idea is confined to these little joys and sorrows and heart-jealousies of the moment. He thinks that this finite thing is the Infinite; and not only so, but he will not let this foolishness go. He clings desperately to trishnā, the thirst after life, what the Buddhists call tanhā and trissā. There may be millions of kinds of happi-

ness and beings and laws and progress and causation,
all acting outside the little universe that we know;
and after all, the whole of this comprises but one
section of our infinite nature.

To acquire freedom we have to get beyond the
limitations of this universe; it cannot be found here.
Perfect equilibrium, or what the Christians call the
peace that passeth all understanding, cannot be had
in this universe, nor in heaven, nor in any place
where our minds and thoughts can go, where the
senses can feel, or of which the imagination can conceive. No such place can give us that freedom, because all such places would be within our universe,
and it is limited by space, time, and causation. There
may be places that are more ethereal than this earth
of ours, where enjoyments are keener; but even those
places must be in the universe, and therefore in
bondage to law. So we have to go beyond, and real
religion begins where this little universe ends. These
little joys and sorrows and this knowledge of things
end there, and Reality begins. Until we give up the
thirst after life, the strong attachment to this our
transient, conditioned existence, we have no hope of
catching even a glimpse of that infinite freedom beyond. It stands to reason then that there is only one
way to attain to that freedom, which is the goal of all
the noblest aspirations of mankind, and that is to give
up this little life, give up this little universe, give up
this earth, give up heaven, give up the body, give up
the mind, give up everything that is limited and conditioned. If we give up our attachment to this little
universe of the senses and of the mind, we shall be

free immediately. The only way to come out of bondage is to go beyond the limitation of law, to go beyond causation.

But it is a most difficult thing to give up the clinging to this universe; few ever attain to that. There are two ways to do it mentioned in our books. One is called "Neti, neti" ("Not this, not this"); the other is called "Iti" ("This"); the former is the negative, and the latter is the positive, way. The negative way is the more difficult. It is only possible for men of the very highest, exceptional minds and gigantic wills, who simply stand up and say, "No, I will not have this," and the mind and body obey their will, and they come out successfully. But such people are very rare. The vast majority of mankind choose the positive way, the way through the world, making use of their bondage in order to break that very bondage. This is also a kind of giving up; only it is done slowly and gradually, by knowing things, enjoying things, and thus obtaining experience and knowing the nature of things until the mind lets them all go at last and becomes unattached. The former way of obtaining non-attachment is by reasoning, and the latter way is through work and experience. The first is the path of jnāna-yoga, characterized by the refusal to do any work; the second is that of karma-yoga, in which there is no cessation from work. Almost everyone in the universe must work. Only those who are perfectly satisfied with the Self, whose desires do not go beyond the Self, whose minds never stray out of the Self, to whom the Self is all in all—only those do not work. The rest must work.

A current of water, rushing down of its own nature, falls into a hollow and makes a whirlpool, and after turning around a little there, it emerges again in the form of the free current to go on unchecked. Each human life is like that current. It gets into the whirl, becomes involved in this world of space, time, and causation, whirls round a little, crying out, "my father, my brother, my name, my fame," and so on, and at last emerges out of it and regains its original freedom. The whole universe is doing that. Whether we know it or not, whether we are conscious or unconscious of it, we are all working to get out of the whirl of the world. The aim of man's experience in the world is to enable him to get out of its whirlpool.

What is karma-yoga? The knowledge of the secret of work. We see that the whole universe is working. For what? For salvation, for liberty. From the atom to the highest being, working for the one end: liberty of the mind, of the body, of the spirit. All things are always trying to get freedom, to fly away from bondage. The sun, the moon, the earth, the planets, all are trying to fly away from bondage. The centrifugal and centripetal forces function throughout the whole universe. Instead of being knocked about in this universe and, after long delay and thrashing, getting to know things as they are, we learn from karma-yoga the secret of work, the method of work, the organizing power of work. A vast mass of energy may be spent in vain if we do not know how to utilize it. Karma-yoga makes a science of work; you learn by it how best to utilize all the activities in this world. Work is inevitable; it must be so. But we should work to the highest purpose. Karma-yoga makes us realize that this world is a world of five minutes, that it is something we have to pass through, and that freedom is not here, but is only to be found beyond. To find the way out of the bondages of the world we have to go through it slowly and surely. There may be exceptional persons, such as those about whom I just spoke, who can stand aside and give up the world as a snake casts off its skin and looks at it as a witness. There are, no doubt, these exceptional beings; but the rest of mankind have to go slowly through this world. Karma-yoga shows the process, the secret and method of doing it to the best advantage.

What does it say? Work incessantly, but give up all attachment to work. Do not identify yourself with anything. Hold your mind free. All that you see, the pains and the miseries, are but the necessary conditions of this world. Poverty and wealth and happiness are but momentary; they do not belong to our real nature at all. Our nature is far beyond misery and happiness, beyond every object of the senses, beyond the imagination. And yet we must go on working all the time. Misery comes through attachment, not through work. As soon as we identify ourselves with the work we do, we feel miserable; but if we do not identify ourselves with it, we do not feel that misery. If a beautiful picture belonging to another is burnt, a man does not generally become miserable; but when his own picture is burnt how miserable he feels! Why? Both were beautiful pictures, perhaps copies of the same original; but in one case very much more misery is felt than in the other. It is because in one case he identifies himself with the picture, and in the other he does not.

This feeling of "I and mine" causes the whole misery. With the sense of possession comes selfishness, and selfishness brings on misery. Every act of selfishness or thought of selfishness makes us attached to something, and immediately we are made slaves. Each wave in the chitta that says "I and mine" immediately puts a chain round us and makes us slaves; and the more we say "I and mine," the more the slavery grows, the more the misery increases. Therefore karma-yoga tells us to enjoy the beauty of all the pictures in the world, but not to identify ourselves with any of them. Never say "mine." Whenever we say a thing is ours, misery immediately comes. Do not say "my child" even in your mind. If you do, then will come misery. Do not say "my house," do not say "my body." The whole difficulty is there. The body is neither yours, nor mine, nor anybody's. These bodies are coming and going by the laws of nature, but the Soul is free, standing as the witness. This body is no more free than a picture or a wall. Why should we be attached so much to a body? Suppose somebody paints a picture; why should he be attached to it? He will have to part with it at death. Do not project that tentacle of selfishness, "I must possess it." As soon as that is done, misery will begin.

So karma-yoga says: First destroy the tendency to project this tentacle of selfishness, and when you have the power of checking it, hold it in and do not allow the mind to get into the wave of selfishness. Then you may go out into the world and work as much as you like. Mix everywhere; go where you please; you will never be contaminated by evil. There is the lotus leaf in the water; the water cannot moisten or stick to it; so will you live in the world. This is called vairāgya, "dispassion" or "non-attachment." I believe I have told you that without non-attachment there cannot be any kind of yoga. Non-attachment is the basis of all the yogas. The man who gives up living in houses, wearing fine clothes, and eating good food, and goes into the desert, may be a most attached person. His only possession, his own body, may become everything to him; and while he lives he will struggle day and night to preserve his body. Non-attachment does not mean anything that we may do in relation to our external body; it is all in the mind. The binding link of "me and mine" is in the mind. If we have not this link with the body and with the things of the senses, we are non-attached, wherever and whatever we may be. A man may be on a throne and perfectly non-attached; another man may be in rags and still very much attached. First we have to attain this state of non-attachment, and then we have to work incessantly. Karma-yoga teaches us the method that will help us in giving up all attachment, though it is indeed very hard.

Here are the two ways of giving up all attachment. One way is for those who do not believe in God or in any outside help. They are left to their own devices; they have simply to work with their own will, with the powers of their mind and discrimination, thinking, "I must be non-attached." For those who believe in God there is another way, which is much less difficult. They give up the fruits of work unto the Lord; they work but never feel attached to the results. Whatever they see, feel, hear, or do is for Him. Whatever good work we may do, let us not claim any praise or benefit for it. It is the Lord's; give up the fruits unto Him. Let us stand aside and think that we are only servants obeying the Lord, our Master, and that every impulse for action comes from Him every moment. Whatever worship you offer, whatever you perceive, whatever you do—give up all unto Him and be at rest. Let us give up our whole body and mind and everything as an eternal sacrifice unto the Lord and be at peace, perfect peace, with ourselves. Instead of pouring oblations into the fire, as in a sacrifice, perform this one great sacrifice day and night—the sacrifice of your little self. "I searched for wealth in this world; Thou art the only wealth I have found; I sacrifice myself unto Thee. I searched for someone to love; Thou art the only beloved I have found; I sacrifice myself unto Thee." Let us repeat this day and night, and say: "Nothing for me. No matter whether the thing is good, bad, or indifferent, I do not care for it. I sacrifice all unto Thee." Day and night let us renounce our seeming self until renunciation becomes a habit with us, until it gets into the blood, the nerves, and the brain, and the whole body is every moment obedient to this idea of self-renunciation. Go then into the battlefield, amidst the roaring cannon and the din of war, and you will find yourself free and at peace.

Karma-yoga teaches us that the ordinary idea of duty is on the lower plane; nevertheless all of us have to do our duty. Yet we may see that this peculiar sense of duty is very often a great cause of misery. Duty becomes a disease with us; it drags us on for ever. It catches hold of us and makes our whole life miserable. It is the bane of human life. This duty, this idea of duty, is the midday summer sun, which scorches the innermost soul of mankind. Look at those poor slaves to duty! Duty leaves them no time to say prayers, no time to bathe; duty is ever on them. They go out and work; duty is on them. They come home and think of the work for the next day; duty is on them. It is living a slave's life, and at last dropping down in the street and dying in harness, like a horse. This is duty as it is understood. The only true duty is to be unattached and to work as free beings, to give up all work unto God. All our duties are His. Blessed are we that we are sent here. We serve our time; whether we do it ill or well, who knows? If we do it well, we shall not think of the fruits. If we do it ill, we shall not worry. Let us be at rest, be free, and work. This kind of freedom is very hard to attain. How easy it is to interpret slavery as duty— the morbid attachment of flesh for flesh as duty! Men go out into the world and struggle and fight for money or for some other thing. Ask them why they do it, and they will say, "It is my duty." But it is only the absurd greed for gold and gain, and they try to cover it with a few flowers.

What is this duty after all? It is really attachment —the impulsion of the flesh. And when an attachment has become established, we call it duty. For instance, where there is no marriage, there is no duty between husband and wife. When marriage comes, husband and wife live together on account of attachment; and that kind of living together becomes accepted after generations; and when it becomes so accepted, it becomes a duty. It is, so to say, a sort of chronic disease. When attachment becomes chronic, we baptize it with the high-sounding name of duty. We strew flowers upon it, trumpets sound for it, and sacred texts are said over it. The whole world fights and men earnestly rob each other for this duty's sake.

Duty is good to the extent that it checks brutality. To the lowest kinds of men, who cannot have any other ideal, it is of some good; but those who want to be karma-yogis must throw this idea of duty overboard. There is no duty for you and me. Whatever you have to give to the world do give by all means, but not as a duty. Do not take any more thought of it. Be not compelled. Why should you be compelled? Everything that you do under compulsion goes to build up attachment. Why should you have any duty? Resign everything unto God. In this tremendous fiery furnace where the fire of duty scorches everybody, drink this nectar of resignation and be happy. We are all simply working out His will and have nothing to do with rewards and punishments. If you want the reward you must also have the punishment; the only way to get out of the punishment is to give up the reward. The only way to get out of misery is to give up the idea of happiness, because

these two are linked to each other. On one side there
is happiness; on the other there is misery. On one
side there is life; on the other there is death. The
only way to get beyond death is to give up the love
of life. Life and death are the same thing looked
at from different points. So the idea of happiness
without misery, or of life without death, is very good
for schoolboys and children; but the thinker sees that
it is all a contradiction in terms and gives up both.
Seek no praise, no reward, for anything you do. No
sooner do we perform a good action than we begin to
desire credit for it. No sooner do we give money to
some charity than we want to see our names blazoned
in the papers. Misery must come as the result of such
desires.

The greatest men in the world have passed away
unknown. The Buddhas and the Christs that we
know are but second-rate heroes in comparison with
the greatest men, of whom the world knows nothing.
Hundreds of these unknown heroes have lived in
every country, working silently. Silently they live
and silently they pass away; and in time their thoughts
find expression in Buddhas or Christs, and it is these
latter who become known to us. The highest men
do not seek any name or fame from their knowledge.
They leave their ideas to the world; they put forth
no claims for themselves and establish no schools or
systems in their name. Their whole nature shrinks
from such a thing. They are the pure sāttvikas, who
never make any stir but only melt down in love. I
have seen one such yogi,[1] who lives in a cave in

[1] A reference to Pavhari Baba.

India. He is one of the most wonderful men I have ever seen. He has so completely lost the sense of his own individuality that we may say that the man in him is entirely gone, leaving behind only the all-comprehending sense of the Divine. If an animal bites one of his arms, he is ready to give it his other arm also and say that it is the Lord's will. Everything that comes to him is from the Lord. He does not show himself to men, and yet he is a magazine of love and of true and sweet ideas.

Next in order come the men with more rajas, or activity—combative natures, who take up the ideas of the perfect ones and preach them to the world. The highest men silently collect true and noble ideas, and others—the Buddhas and the Christs—go from place to place preaching them and working for them. In the life of Gautama Buddha we notice his constantly saying that he is the twenty-fifth Buddha. The twenty-four before him are unknown to history, although the Buddha known to history must have built upon foundations laid by them. The highest men are calm, silent, and unknown. They are the men who really know the power of thought; they are sure that even if they go into a cave and close the door and simply think five true thoughts and then pass away, those five thoughts of theirs will live through eternity. Indeed, such thoughts will penetrate through the mountains, cross the oceans, and travel through the world. They will enter deep into human hearts and brains and raise up men and women who will give them practical expression in the workings of human life. These sāttvika men are too near the Lord to be active and to fight, to be working, struggling, preaching, and doing good to humanity, as they say, here on earth. The active workers, however good, have still a little remnant of ignorance left in them. Only while our nature has yet some impurities left in it can we work. It is in the nature of work to be impelled ordinarily by motive and by attachment. In the presence of an ever active Providence, who notices even the sparrow's fall, how can man attach any importance to his own work? Is it not blasphemy to do so when we know that He is taking care of the minutest things in the world? We have only to stand in awe and reverence before Him, and say, "Thy will be done."

The highest men cannot work, for in them there is no attachment. Those who rejoice in the Self and are satisfied with the Self and are content in the Self alone—for them there is no work to do. Such are indeed the highest among men; but apart from them everyone has to work. In working we should never think that we can help even the least thing in this universe. We cannot. We only help ourselves in this gymnasium of the world. This is the proper attitude for work. If we work in this way, if we always re-member that our present opportunity to work thus is a privilege which has been given to us, we shall never be attached to anything. Millions like you and me think that we are great people in the world; but we all die and in five minutes the world forgets us. But the life of God is infinite. "Who can live a moment, breathe a moment, if this All-powerful One does not will it?" He is the ever active Providence.

All power is His and within His command. Through His command the winds blow, the sun shines, the earth moves, and death stalks upon the earth. He is the All in all; He is all and in all. We can only worship Him. Give up all fruits of work; do good for its own sake; then alone will come perfect non-attachment. The bonds of the heart will thus break, and we shall realize perfect freedom. This freedom is indeed the goal of karma-yoga.

THE IDEAL OF KARMA-YOGA

THE GRANDEST IDEA in the religion of Vedānta is that we may reach the same goal by different paths; and these paths I have generalized into four, namely, those of work, love, psychology, and knowledge. But you must remember, at the same time, that these divisions are not well marked and quite exclusive of each other. Each blends into the other. It is not a fact that you can find men who have no other faculty than that of work, or that you can find men who are devoted worshippers only, or that there are men who cultivate nothing but knowledge. These divisions are made in accordance with the type or the tendency that may be seen to prevail in a man. We have found that, in the end, all these four paths converge and become one. All religions and all spiritual disciplines lead to one and the same goal.

I have already tried to point out that goal. It is, as I understand it, freedom. Everything that we perceive around us is struggling towards freedom, from the atom to man, from the insentient, lifeless particle of matter to the highest existence on earth, the human soul. The world process in fact reveals this struggle for freedom. In all combinations every particle is trying to go its own way, to fly from the other particles; but the others are holding it in check. Our earth is trying to fly away from the sun, and the moon from the earth. Everything has a tendency to infinite dispersion. All that we see in the universe has for its basis this one struggle towards freedom. It is under the impulse of this tendency that the saint prays and the robber robs. When the line of action taken is not a proper one we call it evil, and when the manifestation of it is proper and high we call it good. But the impulse is the same: the struggle towards freedom. The saint is oppressed with the knowledge of his bondage, and he wants to get rid of it; so he worships God. The thief is oppressed with the idea that he does not possess certain things, and he tries to get rid of that want, to obtain freedom from it; so he steals. Freedom is the one goal of all nature, sentient or insentient. And, consciously or unconsciously, everything is struggling towards that goal. The freedom which the saint seeks is very different from that which the robber seeks; the freedom loved by the saint leads him to the enjoyment of infinite, unspeakable bliss, while that on which the robber has set his heart only forges other bonds for his soul.

There is to be found in every religion the manifestation of this struggle towards freedom. It is the groundwork of all morality, of unselfishness, which means getting rid of the idea that men are the same as their little bodies. When we see a man doing good work, helping others, we know that he cannot be confined within the limited circle of "me and mine." There is no limit to this getting out of selfishness. All the great systems of ethics preach absolute unselfishness as the goal. Supposing this absolute unselfishness can be reached by a man, what becomes of him? He is no more the little Mr. So-and-so; he has acquired infinite expansion. That little personality which he had before is now lost to him for ever; he has become infinite; and the attainment of this infinite expansion is indeed the goal of all religions and of all moral and philosophical teachings. The personalist, when he hears this idea expressed philosophically, feels frightened. At the same time, if he preaches morality, he after all teaches the very same idea himself. He puts no limit to the unselfishness of man. Suppose a man becomes perfectly unselfish under the personalistic system, how are we to distinguish him from the perfected ones of other systems? He has become one with the universe, and to become that is the goal of all; only the poor personalist has not the courage to follow out his own reasoning to its right conclusion. Karma-yoga is the attaining through unselfish work of that freedom which is the goal of all human nature. Every selfish action, therefore, retards our reaching the goal, and every unselfish action takes us towards the goal. That is why the only definition that can be given of morality is this: That which is selfish is immoral, and that which is unselfish is moral.

But if you come to details, you will see that the matter is not quite so simple. For instance, as I have already mentioned, environment often makes the details different. The same action under one set of circumstances may be unselfish, and under another set quite selfish. So we can give only a general definition and must leave the details to be worked out by taking into consideration the differences in time, place, and circumstances. In one country one kind of conduct is considered moral, and in another the very same is immoral, because the circumstances differ. The goal of all nature is freedom, and freedom is to be attained only by perfect unselfishness; every thought, word, or deed that is unselfish takes us towards the goal, and as such is called moral. That definition, you will find, holds good in every religion and every system of ethics. In some religious systems, morality is derived from a superior Being—God. If you ask the followers of these systems why a man ought to do this and not that, their answer is: "Because such is the command of God." But whatever be the source from which it is derived, their code of ethics also has the same central idea—not to think of self but to give up self.

And yet some persons, in spite of professing this high ethical idea, are frightened at the thought of having to give up their little personalities. We may ask those who cling to the idea of little personalities to consider the case of a person who has become perfectly unselfish, who has no thought for himself, who does no deed for himself, who speaks no word for himself—and then to say where his "himself" is. That "himself" is known to him only so long as he thinks, acts, or speaks for himself. If he is only conscious of others, of the universe, and of all, where is his "himself"? It is gone for ever.

Karma-yoga, therefore, is a system of discipline aiming at the attainment of freedom through unselfishness and good works. The karma-yogi need not believe in any religious doctrine whatever. He need not believe even in God, may not ask what his soul is or think of any metaphysical speculation. He has his own special aim of realizing selflessness; and he has to work it out himself. Every moment of his life must be realization, because he has to solve by mere work, without the help of doctrine or theory, the very same problem to which the jnāni applies his reason and inspiration and the bhakta his love.

Now comes the next question: What is this work? What is this doing good to the world? Can we do good to the world? In an absolute sense, no; in a relative sense, yes. No permanent or everlasting good can be done to the world; if it could be done, the world would not be this world. We may satisfy the hunger of a man for five minutes, but he will be hungry again. Every pleasure with which we supply a man may be seen to be momentary. No one can permanently cure this ever recurring fever of pleasure and pain. Can any permanent happiness be given to the world? In the ocean a wave cannot arise without causing a hollow somewhere else. The sum total of the good things in the world has been the same throughout in its relation to man's need. It cannot be increased or decreased. Take the history of the human race, as we know it today. Do we not always find the same miseries and the same happinesses, the same pleasures and pains, the same differences in position? Are not some rich, some poor, some high, some low, some healthy, some unhealthy? All this was just the same with the Egyptians, the Greeks, and the Romans in ancient times as it is with the Americans today. So far as history is known, it has always been the same. Yet at the same time we find that along with all these incurable differences of pleasure and pain there has ever been the struggle to alleviate them. Every period of history has given birth to thousands of men and women who have worked hard to smooth the passage of life for others. And how far have they succeeded? We can only play at driving the ball from one place to another. We take away pain from the physical plane and it goes to the mental one. It is like that picture in Dante's hell where the misers were given a mass of gold to roll up a hill. Every time they rolled it up a little, it rolled down again. All our discussions of the millennium are very nice as schoolboys' stories, and they are no better than that. All nations that dream of the millennium also think that they, of all the peoples in the world, will then have the best of it for themselves. This is the wonderfully unselfish idea of the millennium.

We cannot add happiness to this world; similarly, we cannot add pain to it either. The sum total of pleasure and pain displayed here on earth will be the same throughout. We just push it from this side to the other side, and from that side to this; but it will remain the same, because to remain so is its very nature. This ebb and flow, this rising and falling, is in the world's very nature; it would be as logical to hold otherwise as to say that we may have life without death. This is complete nonsense, because the very idea of life implies death and the very idea of pleasure implies pain. The lamp is constantly burning out, and that is its life. If you want to have life you have to die every moment. Life and death are only different expressions of the selfsame thing; they are the same thing looked at from different standpoints; they are the rising and the falling of the same wave, and the two form one whole. One looks at the "fall" side and becomes a pessimist; another looks at the "rise" side and becomes an optimist. When a boy is going to school and his father and mother are taking care of him, everything seems blessed to him; his wants are simple; he is a great optimist. But the old man, with his varied experience, becomes calmer and is sure to have his warmth considerably cooled down. So old nations, with signs of decay all around them, are apt to be less hopeful than new nations. There is a proverb in India: "A thousand years a city, and a thousand years a forest." This change of city into forest and vice versa is going on everywhere, and it makes people optimists or pessimists according to the side they see of it.

The next idea we take up is that of equality. The idea of the millennium has been a great incentive for work. Many religions preach this as one of their ideals —that God is coming to rule the universe and that then there will be no difference at all among men. The people who preach this doctrine are mere fanatics, and fanatics are indeed the sincerest of mankind. Christianity was preached precisely on the basis of the fascination of this fanaticism, and that is what made it so attractive to the Greek and Roman slaves. They believed that under this millennial religion there would be no more slavery, that there would be plenty to eat and drink; and therefore they flocked round the Christian standard. Those who preached the idea were of course ignorant fanatics, but very sincere. In modern times this millennial aspiration is voiced through the slogans of liberty, equality, and fraternity. This also is fanaticism. True equality has never been and never can be on earth. How can we all be equal here? This impossible kind of equality implies total death. What makes this world what it is? Lost balance. In the primal state, which is called chaos, there was perfect balance. How, then, do you explain the diverse forces in the universe? Through struggle, competition, conflict. Suppose that all the particles of matter were held in equilibrium; would there be then any process of creation? We know from science that it is impossible. Disturb a sheet of water, and you will find every particle of the water trying to become calm again, one rushing towards another; and in the same way all the phenomena which we call the universe—all things therein—are struggling to get back to the state of perfect balance. Again a disturbance comes, and again we have combination and creation. Inequality is the very basis of creation. At the same time, the forces struggling to obtain equality are as much a necessity for creation as those which destroy it.

Absolute equality, which means a perfect balance of all the struggling forces in all the planes, can never be had in this world. Before you attain that state, the world will have become quite unfit for any kind of life, and no one will be here. We find, therefore, not only that all these ideas of the millennium and of absolute equality are impossible, but also that, if we try to carry them out, they will surely lead us to the day of destruction. What makes the difference between man and man? It is largely the difference in the brain. Nowadays no one but a lunatic will say that we are all born with the same brain-power. We come into the world with unequal endowments; we come as greater men or as lesser men, and there is no getting away from that pre-natally determined condition. The American Indians were in this country for thousands of years, and a mere handful of your ancestors came to their land. What a difference they have caused in the appearance of the country! Why did not the Indians make improvements and build cities, if all were equal? With your ancestors a different sort of brain-power came into the land; different bundles of past impressions came, and they manifested themselves. Absolute non-differentiation is death. So long as this world lasts, differentiation there will and must be, and the millennium of perfect equality will come only when a cycle of creation comes to its end. Before that, equality cannot be. Yet this idea of realizing the millennium is a great incentive. Just as inequality is necessary for creation, so the struggle to limit it is also necessary. If there were no struggle to become free and return to God, there would be no creation either. It is the difference between these two forces that determines the nature of the motives of men. There will always be these motives for work, some tending towards bondage and others towards freedom.

This world's wheels within wheels are a terrible mechanism. As soon as we put our hands in it, we are caught and we are gone. We all think that when we have done a certain duty we shall be at rest; but before we have done a part of that duty another is already waiting. We are all being dragged along by this mighty, complex world-machine. There are only two ways out of it. One is to give up all concern with the machine and stand aside—that is, to give up all desires. That is very easy to say, but almost impossible to do. I do not know whether in twenty millions of men one can do that. The other way is to plunge into the world and learn the secret of work, and that is the way of karma-yoga. Do not fly away from the wheels of the world-machine, but stand inside it and learn the secret of work. Through proper work done inside, it is also possible to come out. Through this machine itself is the way out.

We have now seen what work is. It is a part of nature's scheme, and it goes on always. Those who believe in God understand this better, because they know that God is not such an incapable being as will need our help. Although this world will go on always, we must remember that our goal is freedom; and according to karma-yoga that goal is to be reached through work. All ideas of making the world perfectly happy may be good as motives for fanatics; but we must know that fanaticism brings forth as much evil as good. The karma-yogi asks why you require any motive for work other than the inborn love of freedom. Go beyond the so-called "worthy" motives. "To work you have the right, but not to the fruits thereof." Man can train himself to know and to practise that, says the karma-yogi. When the idea of doing good becomes a part of his very being, then he will not seek any motive from outside. Let us do good because it is good to do good; he who does good work even in order to get to heaven binds himself down, says the karma-yogi. Any work that is done with even the least selfish motive, instead of making us free, forges one more chain for our feet.

So the only way is to give up all the fruits of work, to be unattached to them. Know that this world is not we, nor are we this world; that we are really not the body; that we really do not work. We are the Self, eternally at rest and at peace. Why should we be bound by anything? It is very good to say that we should be perfectly non-attached; but what is the way to be so? Every good work we do without any ulterior motive, instead of forging a new link will break one of the links in the existing chain. Every good thought we send to the world, without thinking of any return, will be stored up and break one link in the chain, and make us purer and purer, until we become the purest of mortals. Yet all this may seem to be rather quixotic and too philosophical, more theoretical than practical. I have read many arguments against the teachings of the Bhagavad Gītā, and many have said that without motives men cannot work. They have never seen unselfish work except under the influence of fanaticism, and therefore they speak in that way.

Let me tell you in conclusion a few words about one man who actually carried this teaching of karma-yoga into practice. That man is Buddha. He is the one man who has carried it into perfect practice. All the prophets of the world, except Buddha, had external motives to move them to unselfish action. The prophets of the world, with this single exception, may be divided into two groups, one holding that they are Incarnations of God come down on earth, and the other holding that they are Messengers from God; and both draw their impetus for work from outside and expect reward from outside, however highly spiritual may be the language they use. But Buddha is the only prophet who said: "I do not care to know your various theories about God. What is the use of discussing all the subtle doctrines about the soul? Do good and be good, and this will take you to freedom and to whatever truth there is." He was, in the conduct of his life, absolutely without personal motives; and what man worked more than he? Show me one character in history who has soared so high above all. The whole human race has produced but one such character, such high philosophy, such wide sympathy. This great philosopher preached the highest philosophy, and yet had the deepest sympathy for the lowest of animals and never put forth any claims for himself. He is the ideal karma-yogi, acting entirely without motive, and the history of humanity shows him to have been the greatest man ever born —beyond compare the greatest combination of heart and brain that ever existed, the greatest soul-power that has ever been manifested. He is the greatest reformer the world has seen. He was the first who dared to say: "Believe not because some old manuscripts are quoted; believe not because it is your national belief, because you have been made to believe it from your childhood; but reason it all out, and after you have analysed it and found out that it will do good to one and all, then believe it, live up to it, and help others to live up to it."

He works best who works without any motive— neither for money, nor for fame, nor for anything else. And when a man can do that, he will be a Buddha and out of him will come the power to work in such a manner as will transform the world. This man represents the very highest ideal of karma-yoga.

BHAKTI-YOGA

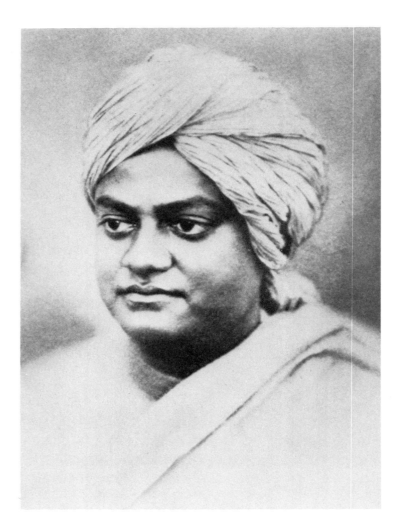

Vivekananda

INVOCATION

"He is the Soul of the universe. He is the Immortal. His is the Rulership. He is the All-knowing, the All-pervading, the Protector of the universe, the Eternal Ruler. None else is there efficient to govern the world eternally.

"He who at the beginning of creation projected Brahmā and who delivered the Vedas unto Him— seeking liberation, I go for refuge unto that Effulgent One, whose light turns the understanding towards the Ātman."—*Śvetāśvatara Upanishad* VI. 17-18.

DEFINITION OF BHAKTI

BHAKTI-YOGA is a real, genuine search after the Lord, a search beginning, continuing, and ending in love. One single moment of the madness of extreme love of God brings us eternal freedom. "Bhakti is intense love of God," says Nārada in his bhakti aphorisms. "When a man gets it he loves all, hates none; he becomes satisfied for ever." "This love cannot be reduced to any earthly benefit"—because so long as worldly desires last that kind of love does not arise. "Bhakti is greater than karma, greater than jnāna, and greater than yoga," because these have in view the attainment of an object, while bhakti is its own fruition, "its own means, and its own end."

Bhakti has been the one constant theme of our sages. Apart from the special writers on bhakti such as Sāndilya or Nārada, the great commentators on the *Vyāsa Sutras*, evident advocates of jnāna, have also something very suggestive to say about love. Even when those commentators are anxious to explain many, if not all, of the texts so as to make them impart a sort of dry knowledge, the sutras, in the chapter on worship especially, do not lend themselves to be easily manipulated in that fashion.

There is not really so much difference between jnāna and bhakti as people sometimes imagine. We shall see, as we go on, that in the end they converge and finally meet in the same point. So also is it with rāja-yoga, which, when pursued as a means to attain liberation and not (as unfortunately it has frequently become in the hands of charlatans and mystery-mongers) as an instrument to hoodwink the unwary, leads us to the same goal.

The one great advantage of bhakti is that it is the easiest and the most natural way to reach the great divine end in view. Its great disadvantage is that in its lower forms it oftentimes degenerates into hideous fanaticism. The fanatical crew in Hinduism or Mohammedanism or Christianity have always been almost exclusively recruited from these worshippers on the lower planes of bhakti. That singleness of attachment (nishthā) to a loved object, without which no genuine love can grow, is very often also the cause of the denunciation of everything else. All the weak and undeveloped minds in every religion or country have only one way of loving their own ideal, and that is to hate every other ideal. Herein is the explanation of why the same man who is so lovingly attached to his own ideal of God, so devoted to his own ideal of religion, becomes a howling fanatic as soon as he sees or hears anything of any other ideal. This kind of love is somewhat like the canine instinct of guarding the master's property from intruders; only the instinct of the dog is better than the reason of man, for the dog never mistakes its master for an enemy, in whatever dress he may come before it. Again, the fanatic loses all power of judgement. Personal considerations are in his case of such absorbing interest that to him it is no question at all of what a man says—whether it is right or wrong; but the one thing he is always particularly careful to know is, who says it. The same man who is kind, good, honest, and loving to people of his own opinion will not hesitate to do the vilest deeds against persons beyond the pale of his own religious brotherhood.

But this danger exists only in that stage of bhakti which is called the gauni or preparatory stage. When bhakti has become ripe and has passed into that form which is called the parā or supreme, no more is there any fear of these hideous manifestations of fanaticism. That soul which is overpowered by this higher form of bhakti is too near the God of Love to become an instrument for the diffusion of hatred.

It is not given to all of us to be harmonious in the building up of our characters in this life; yet we know that that character is of the noblest type in which all these three—knowledge and love and rāja-yoga—are harmoniously fused. Three things are necessary for a bird to fly: the two wings, and the tail as a rudder for steering. Jnāna is the one wing, bhakti is the other, and rāja-yoga is the tail that maintains the balance. For those who cannot pursue all these three forms of worship together in harmony, and take up, therefore, bhakti alone as their way, it is necessary always to remember that forms and ceremonials, though absolutely necessary for the progressing soul, have no other value than to lead us on to that state in which we feel the most intense love of God.

There is a little difference in opinion between the teachers of knowledge and those of love, though both admit the power of bhakti. The jnānis hold bhakti to be an instrument of liberation; the bhaktas look upon it as both the instrument and the thing to be attained. To my mind this is a distinction without much difference. In fact, bhakti, when used as an instrument, really means a lower form of worship; and when this lower form is further cultivated it becomes inseparable from the higher form of bhakti. Each seems to lay great stress upon his own peculiar method of discipline, forgetting that with perfect love true knowledge is bound to come unsought, and that, at the end, true love is inseparable from perfect knowledge.

Bearing this in mind, let us try to understand what the great Vedāntic commentators have to say on the subject. In explaining an aphorism of the *Vedānta Sutras,* Śankara says: "Thus people say, 'He is devoted to the king' or 'He is devoted to the guru.' They say this of him who follows his king or his guru, and does so, having that following as the one end in view. Similarly they say, 'The loving wife meditates on her loving husband away in a foreign land.' Here also a kind of eager and continuous remembrance is meant." This is devotion according to Śankara.

Bhagavān Rāmānuja, in his commentary on the first aphorism of the *Vedānta Sutras,* says:

"Meditation, again, is a constant remembrance [of the thing meditated upon], flowing like an unbroken stream of oil poured from one vessel to another. When this kind of remembering has been attained [in relation to God], all bondages break. Thus it is said in the scriptures regarding constant remembering as a means to liberation. This remembering, again, is of the same form as seeing, because it has the same meaning, as in the passage: 'When He who is far and near is seen, the bonds of the heart are broken, all doubts vanish, and all effects of work disappear.' He who is near can be seen, but he who is far can only be remembered. Nevertheless the scriptures say that we have to see Him who is near as well as far, thereby indicating to us that the above kind of remembering is as good as seeing. This remembrance, when exalted, assumes the same form as seeing. . . . Worship is constant remembering, as may be seen from the principal texts of the scriptures. Knowing, which is the same as repeated worship, has been described as constant remembering. . . . Thus the memory which has attained to the height of what is as good as direct perception is spoken of in the Śruti as a means of liberation. 'This Ātman is not to be reached through various sciences, nor by intellect, nor by much study of the Vedas. Whomsoever this Ātman desires—by him is Ātman attained; unto him Ātman reveals Itself.' Here, after saying that mere hearing, thinking, and meditating are not the means of attaining this Ātman, the Śruti says: 'Whomsoever this Ātman desires—by him is Ātman attained.' The extremely beloved is desired. He by whom this Ātman is extremely beloved becomes the most beloved of the Ātman. So that this beloved may attain the Ātman, the Lord Himself helps. For it has been said by the Lord: 'Those who are constantly attached to Me and worship Me with love—I give that direction to their will by which they come to Me.' Therefore it is said that he to whom this remembering, which is of the same nature as direct perception, is very dear, because it is dear to the object of such memory perception—he is desired by the Supreme Ātman and by him the Supreme Ātman is attained. This constant remembrance is denoted by the word *bhakti*."

In commenting on the sutra of Patanjali, "Or by the worship of the Supreme Lord," Bhoja says: "Pranidhāna ('worship') is that sort of bhakti in which, without one's seeking results, such as sense enjoyments and so forth, all works are dedicated to the Lord, who is the Teacher of teachers." Bhagavān Vyāsa also, when commenting on the same sutra, defines pranidhāna as "the form of bhakti by which the mercy of the Supreme Lord comes to the yogi and blesses him by granting him his desires." According to Śāndilya, "bhakti is intense love of God." The best idea of bhakti, however, is given by the king of bhaktas, Prahlāda: "May that intense and deathless love which ignorant people have for the fleeting objects of the senses not slip away from my heart as I keep meditating on Thee!"

Love for whom? For the Supreme Lord Iśvara. Love for any other being, however great, cannot be bhakti; for, as Rāmānuja says in his Śri Bhāshya, quoting an ancient āchārya, or great teacher: "From Brahmā to a clump of grass, all things that live in the world are slaves of birth and death caused by karma; therefore they cannot be helpful as objects of meditation, because they are all in ignorance and subject to change." In commenting on the word *anurakti* used by Śāndilya, the commentator Svapneśvara says that it means *anu,* after, and *rakti,* attachment; that is to say, the attachment which comes after the knowledge of the nature and glory of God —else a blind attachment to anyone, such as wife or children, would be bhakti. We plainly see, therefore, that bhakti is a series or succession of mental efforts at religious realization, beginning with ordinary worship and ending in a supreme intensity of love for Iśvara.

THE PHILOSOPHY OF IŚVARA

W HO IS IŚVARA? "From whom are the birth, contin-uation, and dissolution of the universe"—He is Iśvara, "the Eternal, the Pure, the Ever Free, the Al-mighty, the All-knowing, the All-merciful, the Teacher of all teachers." And above all, "He is the Lord, whose nature is inexpressible Love."

These certainly are the definitions of a Personal God. Are there then two Gods—the "Not this, not this," the Satchidānanda, the Existence-Knowledge-Bliss, of the philosopher, and this God of Love of the bhakta? No, it is the same Satchidānanda who is also the God of Love—impersonal and personal in one. It has always to be understood that the Personal God worshipped by the bhakta is not separate or different from Brahman. All is Brahman, the One without a second; only Brahman, as Unity or the Absolute, is too much of an abstraction to be loved and wor-shipped. So the bhakta chooses the relative aspect of Brahman, that is, Iśvara, the Supreme Ruler. To use a metaphor: Brahman is the clay or substance out of which an infinite variety of articles are fashioned. As clay, they are all one; but form or manifestation dif-ferentiates one from another. Previously they had all been potentially in the clay; and of course, they are identical in substance. But when formed, and so long as the form remains, they are separate and dif-ferent. The clay mouse can never become a clay elephant, because, as manifestations, form alone

124

makes them what they are, though as unformed clay they are all one. Iśvara, the Personal God, is the highest manifestation of Absolute Reality, or, in other words, the highest possible reading of the Absolute by the human mind. Creation is eternal and so also is Iśvara.

In the fourth pāda of the fourth chapter of his *Sutras*, after saying that almost infinite power and knowledge will come to the liberated soul after the attainment of moksha, Vyāsa states, in an aphorism, that none, however, will get the power of creating, ruling, and dissolving the universe, because that belongs to God alone. In explaining the sutra it is easy for the dualistic commentators to show how it is ever impossible for a subordinate soul, or jiva, to have the infinite power and total independence of God. The thoroughly dualistic commentator Madhvāchārya deals with this passage in his usual summary method by quoting a verse from the *Varāha Purāna*.

In explaining this aphorism the commentator Rāmānuja says: "This doubt being raised, whether among the powers of the liberated soul is included that unique power of the Supreme One, that is, of creating, ruling, and dissolving the universe, and even the Lordship of all, or whether, without that, the glory of the liberated consists only in the direct perception of the Supreme One, we meet with the following objection: 'It is reasonable that the liberated soul should obtain the Lordship of the universe, because the *Mundaka Upanishad* says (III. i. 3.) that the liberated soul, free from sin, attains extreme sameness, which means that it attains oneness with

the Supreme Spirit. It is further stated elsewhere in
the scriptures that all the desires of the liberated are
realized. Now, this extreme sameness and the realization of all desires are not possible without possession
of the power of ruling the universe, which is the
unique power of the Supreme Spirit. Therefore if it
is said that the liberated soul attains the realization
of all desires and extreme sameness, it must be admitted that it obtains the power of ruling the whole
universe.'

"To this we reply that the liberated soul gets all
the powers except that of ruling the universe. Ruling
the universe means guiding the form and the life
and the desires of all sentient and non-sentient
beings. The liberated soul, from whom all that veils
its true nature has been removed, only enjoys the un-
obstructed perception of Brahman, but does not
possess the power of ruling the universe. This is
proved from the scriptural text: 'From whom all these
things are born, by whom all that are born live, unto
whom they, departing, return—ask about It. That is
Brahman.' If this quality of ruling the universe be
common also to the liberated, then this text would
not apply to Brahman as Its definition; but Brahman
is defined as the Ruler of the universe. It is the un-
common attributes which define a thing. Therefore in
texts like: 'My beloved boy, there existed in the beginning only the One without a second. That saw
and reflected: I will give birth to the many. That
projected heat'; 'Brahman, indeed, alone existed in
the beginning. That One evolved. That projected a
blessed form, the Kshatra. All these gods are Kshatras:

Varuna, Soma, Rudra, Parjanya, Yama, Mrityu, Iśāna'; 'Ātman alone, indeed, existed in the beginning; nothing else vibrated. He thought of projecting the world; He projected the world afterwards'; 'Nārāyana alone existed—neither Brahmā nor Iśāna, nor the Dyāvāprithivi, nor the stars nor water nor fire, nor soma nor the sun. He did not take pleasure in being alone. He, after His meditation, created one daughter and the ten organs,' and so forth, and in others, such as: 'Who living in the earth is separate from the earth, who living in the Ātman,' and so forth —the Śrutis speak of the Supreme One as responsible for the work of ruling the universe. Nor in these descriptions of the ruling of the universe is there any reference to the liberated soul by which such a soul may have the ruling of the universe ascribed to it."

In explaining the next sutra, Rāmānuja says: "If you (the opponent) say it is not so, because there are direct texts in the Vedas in evidence to the contrary, we state in reply that these texts refer to the glories of the liberated dwelling in the spheres of the subordinate deities." This also is an easy solution of the difficulty. Although the system of Rāmānuja admits the unity of the total, within that totality of existence there are, according to him, eternal differences. Therefore, for all practical purposes, this system also being dualistic, it was easy for Rāmānuja to keep the distinction between the personal soul and the Personal God very clear.

We shall now try to understand what Śankara, the great teacher of the Advaita school, has to say on the point. We shall see how the Advaita system main-

tains intact all the hopes and aspirations of the
dualist and at the same time propounds its own solution of the problem in consonance with the high
destiny of humanity. Those who aspire to retain their
individual minds even after liberation, and to remain distinct, will have ample opportunity of realizing their aspirations and will enjoy the blessing of
Brahman with attributes. These are they who have
been spoken of in the *Bhāgavata Purāna* thus: "O
King, such are the glorious qualities of the Lord
that the sages whose only pleasure is in the Self, from
whom all fetters have fallen—even they love the
Omnipresent with a love that is for love's sake."
These are they who are spoken of by Sāmkhya as
merged in nature. After having attained perfection
in this cycle, these souls are born in the next as Lords
of world systems. But none of these ever becomes
equal to Iśvara. Those, however, who attain to that
state where there is neither creation nor created nor
Creator, where there is neither knower nor knowable
nor knowledge, where there is neither "I" nor "thou"
nor "he," where there is neither subject nor object
nor relation ("there, who is seen and by whom?")—
such persons have gone beyond everything, to "where
words cannot go nor mind," gone to that which the
Śrutis declare as "Not this, not this." But for those
who cannot or will not reach this state, there will inevitably remain the triune vision of the one undifferentiated Brahman as nature, soul, and the inter-
penetrating sustainer of both—Iśvara.

So, when Prahlāda forgot himself in meditation on
the Lord, he found neither the universe nor its cause;

all was to him one Infinite, undifferentiated by name and form. But as soon as he remembered that he was Prahlāda, there was the universe before him, and with it the Lord of the universe, "the repository of an infinite number of blessed qualities." So it was with the blessed gopis. So long as they had lost the sense of their own personal identity and individuality, they were all Krishnas, and when they began again to think of Him as the One to be worshipped, then they were gopis, and immediately "unto them appeared Krishna with a smile on His lotus face, clad in yellow robes and adorned with garlands, the veritable conqueror [in beauty] of the god of love." (*Bhāgavata Purāna* X. xxxii. 2.)

Now to go back to our Āchārya Śankara: "Suppose," he says, "some by worshipping Brahman with attributes attain conjunction with the Supreme Ruler, preserving their own minds; is their glory limited or unlimited? This doubt arising, the opponent argues: Their glory should be unlimited, because of the scriptural texts: 'They attain their own Kingdom'; 'To him all the gods offer worship'; and 'Their desires are fulfilled in all the worlds.' As an answer to this, Vyāsa says: 'Without the power of ruling the universe.' Barring the power of creating, ruling, and dissolving the universe, the other powers, such as animā and the rest, are acquired by the liberated. As to ruling the universe, that belongs to the eternally perfect Iśvara. Why? Because He is referred to in all the scriptural texts concerning creation and so forth, and the liberated souls are not mentioned therein in any connexion whatsoever. The Supreme

Lord, indeed, is alone engaged in ruling the universe.
The texts as to creation and so forth all point to
Him. Besides there is given the epithet *ever perfect*.
Also the scriptures say that the powers—such as
animā and the rest—of the liberated are derived
from the search after and the worship of God. Therefore they have no place in the ruling of the universe.
Again, on account of their possessing their own
minds, it is possible that their wills might differ and
that while one desired to create, another might desire
to destroy. The only way of avoiding this conflict
is to make all wills subordinate to some one will.
Therefore the conclusion is that the wills of the liberated are dependent on the will of the Supreme
Ruler."

Bhakti, then, can be directed towards Brahman
only in Its personal aspect. "The ideal of the Un-
manifest is hard to attain for those who are identified with their bodies." Bhakti enables us to float
on smoothly with the current of our nature. True it
is that we cannot have any idea of Brahman which
is not anthropomorphic; but is it not equally true
of everything we know? The greatest psychologist
the world has ever known, Kapila, demonstrated ages
ago that human consciousness is one of the elements
in the make-up of all the objects of our perception
and conception, internal as well as external. So we
see that, beginning with our own bodies and going up
to Iśvara, every object of our perception is this consciousness plus something else, whatever that may
be. And this unavoidable mixture is what we ordinarily think of as reality. Indeed it is, and ever will

be, all of reality that it is possible for the human mind to know. Therefore to say that Iśvara is unreal because He is anthropomorphic is sheer nonsense. It sounds very much like the Occidental squabble on idealism and realism, which fearful-looking quarrel has for its foundation a mere play on the word *real*. The idea of Iśvara covers all the ground denoted and connoted by the word *real*, and Iśvara is as real as anything else in the universe. After all, the word *real* means nothing more than what has just been pointed out. Such is our philosophical conception of Iśvara.

SPIRITUAL REALIZATION: THE AIM
OF BHAKTI-YOGA

To THE BHAKTA these dry details are necessary only
to strengthen his will. Beyond that they are of
no use to him; for he is treading on a path which is
fitted to lead him very soon beyond the hazy and
turbulent regions of reason to the realm of realization. He soon, through the mercy of the Lord, reaches
a plane where pedantic and powerless reason is left
far behind, and the mere intellectual groping through
the dark gives place to the daylight of direct perception. He no longer reasons and believes; he almost
perceives. He no longer argues; he senses. And is not
this seeing God and feeling God and enjoying God
higher than everything else? Nay, bhaktas have not
been wanting who have maintained that it is higher
even than moksha, liberation. And is it not also the
highest utility? There are people in the world—and
a good many of them too—who are convinced that
only that is of use to man which brings him creature
comforts. Even religion, God, eternity, the soul—
none of these is of any use to them, since they do
not bring them money or physical comfort. To such,
all those things which do not go to gratify the senses
and appease the appetites are of no use. In every
mind, utility, however, is conditioned by its own
peculiar wants. To men, therefore, who never rise
higher than eating, drinking, begetting progeny, and
dying, the only gain is in sense enjoyment; and

they must wait and go through many more births and reincarnations to learn to feel even the faintest necessity for anything higher. But those to whom the eternal interests of the soul are of much higher value than the fleeting interests of this mundane life, to whom the gratification of the senses is but the thoughtless play of the baby—to them, God and the love of God form the highest and the only utility of human existence. Thank God, there are some such still living in this world of too much worldliness.

Bhakti-yoga, as we have said, is divided into the gauni or preparatory stage, and the parā or supreme stage. We shall find, as we go on, how in the preparatory stage we unavoidably stand in need of many concrete helps to enable us to make progress. And indeed, the mythological and symbolical parts of all religions are natural growths which early environ the aspiring soul and help it Godward. It is also a significant fact that spiritual giants have been produced only in those systems of religion where there is an exuberant growth of rich mythology and ritualism. The dry, fanatical forms of religion, which attempt to eradicate all that is poetical, all that is beautiful and sublime, all that gives a firm grasp to the infant mind tottering on its Godward way—the forms which attempt to break down the very ridge-poles of the spiritual roof, and in their ignorant and superstitious conceptions of truth try to drive away all that is life-giving, all that furnishes the formative material to the spiritual plant growing in the human soul—such forms of religion too soon find that all that is left to them is but an empty shell, a contentless

frame of words and sophistry, with perhaps a little
flavour of a kind of social scavengering or the so-
called spirit of reform.

The vast mass of those whose religion is like this
are conscious or unconscious materialists—the aim of
their lives here and hereafter being material enjoyment, which, indeed, is to them the alpha and omega
of human life. Ishtāpurta—work like street-cleaning
and scavengering intended for the material comfort
of man—is, according to them, the be-all and end-
all of human existence. And the sooner the followers
of this curious mixture of ignorance and fanaticism
come out in their true colours and join, as they well
deserve to do, the ranks of atheists and materialists,
the better it will be for the world. One ounce of the
practice of righteousness and of spiritual self-realiza-
tion outweighs tons and tons of frothy talk and
nonsensical sentiments. Show us one, but one, gigantic spiritual genius growing out of all this dry dust
of ignorance and fanaticism; and if you cannot, close
your mouths, open the windows of your hearts to
the clear light of truth, and sit like children at the
feet of those who know what they are talking about
—the sages of India. Let us, then, listen attentively
to what they say.

THE NEED OF A GURU

Every soul is destined to be perfect, and every being, in the end, will attain the state of perfection. Whatever we are now is the result of our acts and thoughts in the past, and whatever we shall be in the future will be the result of what we think and do now. But this, the shaping of our own destinies, does not preclude our receiving help from outside; nay, in the vast majority of cases such help is absolutely necessary. When it comes, the higher powers and possibilities of the soul are quickened, spiritual life is awakened, growth is animated, and in the end man becomes holy and perfect.

This quickening impulse cannot be derived from books. The soul can receive impulses only from another soul, and from nothing else. We may study books all our lives, we may become very intellectual, but in the end we find that spiritually we have not developed at all. It is not true that a high order of intellectual development always goes hand in hand with a proportionate development of the spiritual side in man. In studying books we are sometimes deluded into thinking that thereby we are being spiritually helped; but if we analyse the effect of the study of books on ourselves, we shall find that, at the utmost, it is only our intellect that derives profit from such studies, and not our inner spirit. This inadequacy of books to quicken spiritual growth is the reason why, although almost every one of us can *speak* most wonderfully

on spiritual matters, when it comes to action and the
living of a truly spiritual life, we find ourselves so
awfully deficient. To quicken the spirit, the impulse
must come from another soul.

The person from whose soul such an impulse comes
is called the guru, the teacher; and the person to whose
soul the impulse is conveyed is called the śishya, the
student. To convey such an impulse to any soul, in
the first place, the soul from which it proceeds must
possess the power of transmitting it, as it were, to
another; and in the second place, the soul to which
it is transmitted must be fit to receive it. The seed
must be a living seed, and the field must be ready
ploughed; and when both these conditions are fulfilled
a wonderful growth of genuine religion takes place.
"The true preacher of religion has to be of wonderful
capabilities, and clever shall his hearer be"; and when
both of these are really wonderful and extraordinary,
then will result a splendid spiritual awakening, and
not otherwise. Such alone are the real teachers, and
such alone are also the real students, the real aspirants.
All others are only playing with spirituality. They have
just a little curiosity awakened, just a little intellectual
aspiration kindled in them, and are merely standing
on the outward fringe of the horizon of religion. There
is, no doubt, some value even in that, since it may,
in course of time, result in the awakening of a real
thirst for religion; and it is a mysterious law of nature
that as soon as the field is ready, the seed must and
does come; as soon as the soul earnestly desires to have
religion, the transmitter of the religious force must and
does appear to help that soul. When the power which

attracts the light of religion in the receiving soul is full and strong, the power which answers to that attraction and sends in light does come as a matter of course.

There are, however, certain great dangers in the way. There is, for instance, the danger to the receiving soul of its mistaking momentary emotions for real religious yearning. We may see this in ourselves. Many a time in our lives somebody dies whom we loved. We receive a blow; we feel that the world is slipping between our fingers, that we want something surer and higher, that we must become religious. In a few days that wave of feeling passes away, and we are left stranded exactly where we were before. All of us often mistake such impulses for real thirst after religion; but as long as these momentary emotions are thus mistaken, that continuous, real craving of the soul for religion will not come, and we shall not find the true transmitter of spirituality. So whenever we are tempted to complain that our search after the truth that we desire so much is proving vain—instead of so complaining, our first duty is to look into our own souls and find whether the craving in the heart is real. Then, in the vast majority of cases, it will be discovered that we were not fit to receive the truth, that there was no real thirst for spirituality.

There are still greater dangers in regard to the transmitter, the guru. There are many who, though immersed in ignorance, yet, in the pride of their hearts, fancy they know everything and not only do not stop there, but offer to take others on their shoulders; and thus, the blind leading the blind, both fall into the ditch. "Fools dwelling in darkness, wise in their own conceit and puffed up with vain knowledge, go round and round, staggering to and fro, like blind men led by the blind." (*Mundaka Upanishad* I. ii. 8.) The world is full of these. Everyone wants to be a teacher; every beggar wants to make a gift of a million dollars! Just as such beggars are ridiculous, so are such teachers.

QUALIFICATIONS OF THE ASPIRANT
AND THE TEACHER

How, THEN, are we to know a teacher? The sun requires no torch to make it visible; we need not light a candle in order to see it. When the sun rises, we instinctively become aware of the fact, and when a teacher of men comes to help us, the soul will instinctively know that truth has already begun to shine upon it. Truth stands on its own evidence; it does not require any other testimony to demonstrate it. It is self-effulgent. It penetrates into the innermost corners of our nature, and in its presence the whole universe stands up and says, "This is truth." Those teachers whose wisdom and truth shine like the light of the sun are the very greatest the world has known, and they are worshipped as God by the major portion of mankind. But we may get help from comparatively lesser teachers also; only we ourselves do not possess intuition enough to judge properly of the man from whom we receive teaching and guidance. So there ought to be certain tests, certain conditions, for the teacher to satisfy, as also for the taught.

The conditions necessary for the taught are purity, a real thirst after knowledge, and perseverance. No impure soul can be really religious. Purity in thought, speech, and act is absolutely necessary for anyone to be religious. As to the thirst after knowledge, it is an old law that we all get only what we want. None of us can get anything other than what we fix our hearts upon. To pant for religion is truly a very difficult thing; it is not as easy as we generally imagine. Hearing religious talks, reading religious books, is no proof yet of a real want felt in the heart. There must be a continuous struggle, a constant fight, an unremitting grappling with our lower nature, till the higher want is actually felt and the victory is achieved. It is not a question of one or two days, of years, or of lives; the struggle may have to go on for hundreds of lifetimes. Success may sometimes come immediately, but we must be ready to wait patiently even for what may look like an infinite length of time. The student who sets out with such a spirit of perseverance will surely find success and realization at last.

With regard to the teacher, we must see that he knows the spirit of the scriptures. The whole world reads Bibles, Vedas, and Korans; but they are all only words, syntax, etymology, philology—the dry bones of religion. The teacher who deals too much in words and allows the mind to be carried away by the force of words loses the spirit. It is knowledge of the spirit of the scriptures, alone, that characterizes the true religious teacher. The network of the words of the scriptures is like a huge forest, in which the human mind often loses itself and finds no way out. "The network of words is a big forest; it is the cause of aimless wandering of the mind." "The various methods of joining words, the various methods of speaking in beautiful language, the various methods of explaining the diction of the scriptures, are only for the disputations and enjoyment of the learned; they do not conduce to the development of spiritual perception." Those who employ such methods to impart religion to others are only desirous to show off their learning, so that the world may praise them as great scholars. You will find that not one of the great teachers of the world ever went into these various explanations of the texts; there is with them no attempt at "text-torturing," no eternal playing upon the meaning of words and their roots. Yet they taught nobly, while others who have nothing to teach have taken up a word, sometimes, and written a three-volume book on its origin, on the man who used it first, and on what that man was accustomed to eat and how long he slept, and so on.

Bhagavān Ramakrishna used to tell a story about some men who went into a mango orchard and busied themselves in counting the leaves, the twigs, and the branches, examining their colour, comparing their size, and noting down everything most carefully, and who then got up a learned discussion on each of these topics, which were undoubtedly highly interesting to them. But another man, more sensible than they, did not care for all these things and instead began to eat the mangoes. And was he not wise? So leave this counting of leaves and twigs and this note-taking to others. This kind of work has its proper place, but not here in the spiritual domain. You never see a strong spiritual man among these "leaf-counters." Religion, the highest aim, the highest glory of man, does not require so much labour. If you want to be a bhakta, it is not at all necessary for you to know whether Krishna was born in Mathurā or in Vraja, what He did, or the exact date on which He imparted the teachings of the Gītā. You only need to feel the crav-

ing for the beautiful lessons about duty and love in
the Gitā. All the other particulars about it and its
author are for the enjoyment of the learned. Let them
have what they desire. Say, "Śāntih, śāntih!" to their
learned controversies, and you yourself "eat the
mangoes."

The second condition necessary in the teacher is
sinlessness. The question is often asked: "Why should
we look into the character and personality of a
teacher? We have only to judge of what he says and
take that up." This is not right. If a man wants to
teach me something of dynamics or chemistry or any
other physical science, he may be anything he likes,
because what the physical sciences require is merely
an intellectual equipment; but in the spiritual sciences
it is impossible from first to last that there should be
any spiritual light in the soul that is impure. What
religion can an impure man teach? The *sine qua non*
of acquiring spiritual truth for oneself, or for impart-
ing it to others, is purity of heart and soul. A vision of
God or a glimpse of the beyond never comes until the
soul is pure. Hence, with the teacher of religion, we
must see first what he *is* and then what he says. He
must be perfectly pure, and then alone will his words
come to have value, because he is only then a true
transmitter. What can he transmit if he has no spiritual
power in himself? There must be a worthy vibration
of spirituality in the mind of the teacher so that it
may be sympathetically conveyed to the mind of the
taught. The function of the teacher is indeed an affair of the transference of something, and not one of
mere stimulation of the existing intellectual or other

faculties in the taught. Something real and appreciable as an influence comes from the teacher and goes to the taught. Therefore the teacher must be pure.

The third condition is with regard to the motive. The teacher must not teach with any ulterior, selfish motive—for money, name, or fame; his work must be simply out of love, out of pure love for mankind at large. The only medium through which spiritual force can be transmitted is love. Any selfish motive, such as the desire for gain or for name, will immediately destroy this conveying medium. God is love, and only he who has known God as love can be a teacher of godliness and God to man.

When you see that in your teacher these conditions are all fulfilled, you are safe. If they are not, it is unsafe to allow yourself to be taught by him; for there is the great danger that, if he cannot convey goodness to your heart, he may convey wickedness. This danger must by all means be guarded against. "He who is learned in the scriptures, sinless, unpolluted by lust, and is the greatest knower of Brahman" is the real teacher.

From what has been said, it naturally follows that we cannot be taught to love, appreciate, and assimilate religion everywhere, by everybody. "Sermons in stones, books in the running brooks, and good in everything" —is all very true as a poetical figure; but nothing can impart to a man a single grain of truth unless he has the undeveloped germ of it in himself. To whom do the stones and brooks preach sermons? To that human soul the lotus of whose holy inner shrine is already about to open. And the light which causes the beautiful opening of this lotus comes always from the good and wise teacher. When the heart has thus been opened, it becomes fit to receive teaching from the stones or the brooks, the stars or the sun or the moon, or from anything that exists in our divine universe; but the unopened heart will see in them nothing but mere stones or mere brooks. A blind man may go to a museum, but he will not profit by it in any way; his eyes must be opened first, and then alone will he be able to learn what the things in the museum can teach.

This eye-opener of the aspirant after religion is the teacher. With the teacher, therefore, our relationship is the same as that between a descendant and his ancestor. Without faith, humility, submission, and veneration in our hearts towards our religious teacher, there cannot be any growth of religion in us. It is a significant fact that where this kind of relation between the teacher and the taught prevails, there alone do gigantic spiritual men grow, while in those countries which have neglected to keep up this kind of relation, the religious teacher has become a mere lecturer—the teacher expecting his five dollars and the person taught expecting his brain to be filled with the teacher's words, and each going his own way after this much has been done. Under such circumstances spirituality becomes almost an unknown quantity. There is none to transmit it and none to have it transmitted to. Religion with such people becomes a business; they think they can obtain it with their dollars. Would to God that religion could be obtained so easily! But unfortunately it cannot be.

Religion, which is the highest knowledge and the

highest wisdom, cannot be bought, nor can it be acquired from books. You may thrust your head into all the corners of the world, you may explore the Himālayas, the Alps, and the Caucasus, you may sound the bottom of the sea and pry into every nook of Tibet and the desert of Gobi, but you will not find it anywhere until your heart is ready to receive it and your teacher has come. And when that divinely appointed teacher comes, serve him with childlike confidence and simplicity, freely open your heart to his influence, and see in him God manifested. Those who come to seek the truth with such a spirit of love and veneration—to them the Lord of Truth reveals the most wonderful things regarding truth, goodness, and beauty.

INCARNATIONS

Wherever His name is spoken, that very place is holy. How much more so is the man who speaks His name, and with what veneration ought we to approach that man out of whom comes to us spiritual truth! Such great teachers of spiritual truth are indeed very few in number in this world; but the world is never altogether without them. They are always the fairest flowers of human life—"an ocean of mercy without any motive." "Know the guru to be Me," says Śrī Krishna in the *Bhāgavata*. The moment the world is absolutely bereft of these, it becomes a hideous hell and hastens on to its destruction.

Higher and nobler than all ordinary teachers in the world is another set of teachers, the Avatāras of Iśvara. They can transmit spirituality with a touch, even with a mere wish. At their command the lowest and most degraded characters become saints in one second. They are the Teachers of all teachers, the highest manifestations of God through man. We cannot see God except through them. We cannot help worshipping them. And indeed they are the only ones whom we are bound to worship.

No man can really see God except through these human manifestations. If we try to see God otherwise, we make for ourselves a hideous caricature of Him and believe the caricature to be as good as the original. There is a story of an ignorant man who was asked to make an image of the god Śiva, and who, after days of hard struggle, manufactured only the image of a monkey. So whenever we try to think of God as He is in His absolute perfection, we invariably meet with the most miserable failure; because as long as we are men we cannot conceive Him as being anything higher than a man. The time will come when we shall transcend our human nature and know Him as He is; but as long as we are men we must worship Him in man and as a man.

Talk as you may, try as you may, you cannot think of God except as a man. You may deliver great intellectual discourses on God and on all things under the sun, become great rationalists, and prove to your satisfaction that all these accounts of the Avatāras of God as men are nonsense. But let us come for a moment to practical common sense. What is there behind this kind of remarkable intellect? Zero, nothing, simply so much froth. When next you hear a man delivering a great intellectual lecture against this worship of the Avatāras of God, get hold of him and ask him what *his* idea of God is, what he understands by "omnipotence," "omnipresence," and all such terms, beyond the spelling of the words. He really means nothing by them; he cannot formulate as their meaning any idea unaffected by his own human nature. He is no better off in this matter than the man in the street who has not read a single book. That man in the street, however, is quiet and does not disturb the peace of the world, while this big talker creates disturbance and misery among mankind. Religion is, after all, realization, and we must

make the sharpest distinction between talk and in-
tuitive experience. What we experience in the depths
of our souls is realization. Nothing indeed is so un-
common as common sense in regard to this matter.

By our present constitution we are limited and
bound to see God as a man. If, for instance, the buf-
faloes want to worship God, they will, in keeping
with their own nature, see Him as a huge buffalo; if
the fish want to worship God, they will have to form
an idea of Him as a big fish; and men have to think
of Him as a man. And these various conceptions are
not due to a morbidly active imagination. Man, buffalo, and fish all may be supposed to represent so
many different vessels, so to say. All these vessels go
to the sea of God to get filled with water, each according to its own shape and capacity. In the man,
the water takes the shape of a man, in the buffalo,
the shape of a buffalo, and in the fish, the shape of a
fish. In each of these vessels there is the same water of
the sea of God. When men see Him, they see Him as
a man, and the animals, if they have any conception
of God at all, must see Him as an animal, each according to his own ideal. So we cannot help seeing God
as a man; and therefore we are bound to worship Him
as a man. There is no other way.

Two kinds of men do not worship God as a man:
the human brute, who has no religion, and the
paramahamsa, who has risen beyond all the weaknesses of humanity and has transcended the limits
of his own human nature. To him all nature has become his own Self. He alone can worship God as
He is. Here too, as in all other cases, the two ex-

tremes meet. The extreme of ignorance and the other extreme of knowledge—neither of these goes through acts of worship. The human brute does not worship because of his ignorance, and the jivanmuktas, the free souls, do not worship because they have realized God in themselves. If anyone between these two poles of existence tells you that he is not going to worship God as a man, kindly beware of that person. He is, not to use any harsher term, an irresponsible talker; his religion is for unsound and empty brains.

God understands human failings and becomes man to do good to humanity. "Whenever virtue subsides and wickedness prevails I manifest Myself. To establish virtue, to destroy evil, to save the good, I embody Myself in every yuga." "Fools deride Me who have assumed the human form, without knowing My real nature as the Lord of the universe." Such is Śri Krishna's declaration, in the Gitā, on the Incarnation. "When a huge tidal wave comes," says Bhagavān Śri Ramakrishna, "all the little brooks and ditches become full to the brim without any effort or consciousness on their own part; so when an Incarnation comes, a tidal wave of spirituality breaks upon the world, and people feel spirituality in the very air."

THE MANTRA: OM

B<small>UT WE ARE</small> now considering not these Mahāpu-
rushas, the great Incarnations, but only the
siddha-gurus, the teachers who have attained the
goal. They, as a rule, have to convey the germs of
spiritual wisdom to the disciple by means of mantras,
or words to be meditated upon. What are these
mantras?

The whole of this universe has, according to Indian
philosophy, both name and form as its conditions of
manifestation. In the human microcosm there cannot
be a single wave in the mind-stuff which is not conditioned by name and form. If it be true that nature
is built throughout on the same plan, this kind of
conditioning by name and form must also be the plan
of the building of the whole of the cosmos. "As, one
lump of clay being known, all things of clay are
known," so the knowledge of the microcosm must
lead to the knowledge of the macrocosm. Now, the
form is the outer crust, and the name or the idea is
the inner essence or kernel. The body is the form, and
the mind, or antahkarana, is the name; and sound-
symbols are universally associated with the names in
all beings having the power of speech. In the individual man the thought-waves rising in the limited
mahat, known as the chitta or mind-stuff, must manifest themselves first as words and then as the more
concrete forms.

In the universe, Brahmā (Hiranyagarbha or the

cosmic mahat) first manifested Himself as name and then as form, that is to say, as this universe. All this expressed, sensible universe is the form, and behind it stands the eternal, inexpressible Sphota, the manifester, as Logos or Word. This eternal Sphota, the essential and eternal material of all ideas or names, is the power through which the Lord creates the universe. Nay, the Lord first becomes conditioned as the Sphota and then evolves Himself as the yet more concrete sensible universe. This Sphota has one word as its only possible symbol, and this is Om. And as we can by no possible means of analysis separate the word from the idea, Om and the eternal Sphota are inseparable; and therefore it is out of this holiest of all holy words, the mother of all names and forms, the eternal Om, that the whole universe may be supposed to have been created.

But it may be said that, although thought and word are inseparable, yet as there may be various word-symbols for the same thought, it is not necessary that this particular word Om should be the word representative of the thought out of which the universe has become manifested. To this objection we reply that this Om is the only possible symbol which covers the whole ground, and there is none other like it. The Sphota is the material of all words; yet it is not any definite word in its fully formed state. That is to say, if all the peculiarities which distinguish one word from another be removed, then what remains will be the Sphota. Therefore this Sphota is called the Nāda-Brahman, the Sound-Brahman. Now, as every word-symbol intended to express the inexpressi-

ble Sphota will so particularize it that it will no longer
be the Sphota, that symbol which particularizes it
the least and at the same time most approximately
expresses its nature will be the truest symbol thereof.
This is Om, and Om only, because these three letters—A, U, M—pronounced in combination as Om,
may well be the generalized symbol of all possible
sounds. The letter A is the least differentiated of all
sounds; therefore Krishna says in the Gitā, "I am A
among the letters." Again, all articulate sounds are
produced in the space within the mouth, beginning
with the root of the tongue and ending in the lips.
The throat sound is A, and M is the last lip sound,
and U exactly represents the rolling forward of the
impulse, which begins at the root of the tongue and
ends in the lips. If properly pronounced, this Om
will represent the whole phenomenon of sound-pro-
duction; and no other word can do this. This, therefore, is the fittest symbol of the Sphota, which is the
real meaning of Om. And as the symbol can never be
separated from the thing signified, Om and the Sphota
are one. Furthermore, as the Sphota, being the finer
side of the manifested universe, is nearer to God and is
indeed the first manifestation of Divine Wisdom, this
Om is the true symbol of God.

Again, just as the non-dual Brahman, the Akhanda
Satchidānanda, the undivided Existence-Knowledge-
Bliss, can be conceived by imperfect human souls only
from particular standpoints and associated with particular qualities, so this universe, Its body, has also to
be thought of according to the particular trend of the
thinker's mind. This direction of the worshipper's

mind is guided by its prevailing elements, or tattvas. As a result, the same Reality will be seen in various manifestations as the possessor of various predominant qualities, and the same universe will appear full of manifold forms. Even as in the case of the least differentiated and most universal symbol Om, thought and sound-symbol are seen to be inseparably associated with each other, so also this law of their inseparable association applies to the many differentiated views of God and the universe. Each of them, therefore, must have a particular word-symbol to express it. These word-symbols, evolved out of the deepest spiritual perceptions of sages, symbolize and express as nearly as possible the particular view of God and the universe they stand for. As Om represents the Akhanda, the undifferentiated Brahman, so the others represent the khanda or differentiated views of the same Being; and they are all helpful to divine meditation and the acquisition of true knowledge.

WORSHIP OF SUBSTITUTES AND IMAGES

THE NEXT POINTS to be considered are the worship of pratikas, or things more or less satisfactory as substitutes for God, and the worship of pratimās, or images. What is the worship of God through a pratika? It means "joining the mind with devotion to what is not Brahman, taking it to be Brahman," says Bhagavān Rāmānuja. Śankara says, "Worship of the mind as Brahman—this is worship with regard to the internal; and of the ākāśa as Brahman—this is with regard to the gods." The mind is an internal pratika; ākāśa is an external one; and both have to be worshipped as substitutes for God. Similarly: " 'The sun is Brahman; this is the command'; 'He who worships name as Brahman'—in all such passages a doubt arises as to the worship of pratikas," says Śankara. The word *pratika* means "going towards"; and worshipping a pratika means worshipping, as a substitute, something which is, in one or more respects, like Brahman, but is not Brahman. Along with the pratikas mentioned in Śruti there are various others to be found in the Purānas and the Tantras. In this kind of pratika-worship may be included all the various forms of pitri-worship and deva-worship.

Now, worshipping Iśvara, and Him alone, is bhakti; the worship of anything else—deva or pitri or any other being—cannot be bhakti. The various kinds of worship of the various devas are all included in ritualistic karma, which gives to the worshipper only a particular result in the form of some celestial enjoyment, but can neither give rise to bhakti nor lead to mukti. One thing therefore has to be carefully borne in mind. If, as it may happen in some cases, the highly philosophic ideal, the Supreme Brahman, is dragged down by pratika-worship to the level of the pratika and the pratika itself is taken to be the Ātman of the worshipper, his Antaryāmin, then the worshipper becomes entirely misled; for no pratika can really be the Ātman of the worshipper. But where Brahman Himself is the object of worship, and the pratika stands only as a substitute or a suggestion thereof, that is to say, where, through the pratika, the omnipresent Brahman is worshipped, the pratika itself being idealized into the cause of all, or Brahman—the worship is positively beneficial. Nay, it is absolutely necessary for all mankind until they have got beyond the primary or preparatory state of the mind with regard to worship.

When, therefore, any gods or other beings are worshipped in and for themselves, such worship is only ritualistic karma; and as a vidyā, a science, it gives us only the fruit belonging to that particular vidyā. But when the devas or any other beings are looked upon as Brahman and worshipped, the result obtained is the same as that obtained by the worshipping of Iśvara.

This explains how in many cases, both in the Śrutis and in the Smritis, a god or a sage or some other extraordinary being is taken up and lifted, as it were, out of his own nature and idealized into Brahman, and is then worshipped. Says the Advaitist, "Is not everything Brahman when the name and the form have been removed from it?" "Is not He, the Lord, the innermost Self of everyone?" says the Viśishtād-vaitist. "The fruition of even the worship of the Ādityas, and so forth, Brahman Himself bestows, because He is the Ruler of all." Says Śankara, in his *Brahma Sutra* Bhāshya: "Here, in this way, Brahman becomes the object of worship, because He, as Brahman, is superimposed on the pratikas, just as Vishnu, and so forth, are superimposed upon images."

The same ideas apply to the worship of the pratimās as to that of the pratikas. That is to say, if the image stands for a god or a saint, the worship does not result in bhakti and does not lead to liberation; but if it stands for the one God, the worship thereof will bring both bhakti and mukti. Of the principal religions of the world, we see Vedānta, Buddhism, and certain forms of Christianity freely using images; only two religions, Mohammedanism and Protestantism, refuse such help. Yet the Mohammedans use the graves of their saints and martyrs almost in the place of images; and the Protestants, in rejecting all concrete helps to religion, are drifting away every year farther and farther from spirituality, till at present there is scarcely any difference between the advanced Protestants and the followers of Auguste Comte, or the agnostics, who preach ethics alone. Again, in Christianity and Mohammedanism whatever exists of image worship is made to fall under that category in which the pratika or the pratimā is worshipped in itself, but not as a help to the vision of God. Therefore it is at best only of the nature of ritualistic karma and cannot produce either bhakti or mukti. In this form of image worship, the allegiance of the soul is given to other things than Iśvara, and therefore such use of images or graves, of temples or tombs, is real idolatry. It is in itself neither sinful nor wicked. It is a rite, a karma, and worshippers must and will get the fruit thereof.

THE CHOSEN IDEAL

THE NEXT THING to be considered is what we know as Ishta-nishthā, or devotion to the "Chosen Ideal." One who aspires to be a bhakta must know that "so many opinions are so many ways." He must know that all the various sects of the different religions are the various manifestations of the glory of the same Lord. "They call You by so many names; they divide You, as it were, by different names; yet in each one of these is to be found Your omnipotence. . . . You reach the worshipper through all of these; there is no special time for Your worship so long as the soul has intense love for You. You are so easy of approach; it is my misfortune that I cannot love You." Not only this. The bhakta must take care not to hate, or even criticize, those radiant sons of light who are the founders of various sects; he must not even hear them spoken ill of.

Very few, indeed, are those who are at once the possessors of an extensive sympathy and power of appreciation as well as of an intense love. We find, as a rule, that liberal and sympathetic sects lose the intensity of religious feeling, and in their hands religion is likely to degenerate into a kind of politico-social club life. On the other hand, intensely narrow sectarians, while displaying a very commendable love for their own ideals, are seen to have acquired every particle of that love by hating everyone who is not of exactly the same opinion as themselves. Would

to God that this world were full of men who were
as intense in their love as they were world-wide in
their sympathies! But such are few and far between.
Yet we know that it is practicable to educate large
numbers of human beings in the ideal of a wonderful blending of both the breadth and the intensity
of love; and the way to do that is by this path of
Ishta-nishthā.

Every sect of every religion presents only one ideal
of its own to mankind; but the eternal Vedāntic religion opens to mankind an infinite number of doors
for ingress into the inner shrine of Divinity, and
places before humanity an almost inexhaustible array
of ideals, there being in each of them a manifestation of the Eternal One. With the kindest solicitude
Vedānta points out to aspiring men and women the
numerous roads hewn out of the solid rock of the
realities of human life by the glorious sons, or human
manifestations, of God in the past and in the present,
and stands with outstretched arms to welcome all
—to welcome even those that are yet to be—to that
Home of Truth and that Ocean of Bliss wherein the
human soul, liberated from the net of māyā, may
transport itself with perfect freedom and with eternal
joy.

Bhakti-yoga, therefore, lays on us the imperative
command not to hate or deny any one of the various
paths that lead to salvation. Yet the growing plant
must be hedged round to protect it until it has grown
into a tree. The tender plant of spirituality will die
if exposed too early to the action of a constant change
of ideas and ideals. Many people, in the name of

what may be called religious liberalism, may be seen
feeding their idle curiosity with a continuous succession of different ideals. With them, hearing new
things grows into a kind of disease, a sort of religious drink-mania. They want to hear new things
just by way of getting a temporary nervous excite-
ment, and when one such exciting influence has had
its effect on them, they are ready for another. Religion is with these people a sort of intellectual opium-
eating, and there it ends. "There is another sort of
man," says Bhagavān Ramakrishna, "who is like the
pearl-oyster of the story. The pearl-oyster leaves its
bed at the bottom of the sea and comes up to the
surface to catch the rain-water when the star Svāti
is in the ascendant. It floats about on the surface of
the sea with its shell wide open until it has succeeded
in catching a drop of the rain-water, and then it dives
deep down to its sea-bed and there rests until it has
succeeded in fashioning a beautiful pearl out of that
raindrop." This is indeed the most poetical and forci-
ble way in which the theory of Ishta-nishthā has ever
been put.

Eka-nishthā, or devotion to one ideal, is absolutely
necessary for the beginner in the practice of religious
devotion. He must say with Hanumān in the
Rāmāyana: "Though I know that the Lord of Śri
and the Lord of Jānaki[1] are both manifestations of
the same Supreme Being, yet my All in all is the
lotus-eyed Rāma." Or, as was said by the sage Tulsidās: "Take the sweetness of all, sit with all, take the
name of all, say yea, yea—but keep your seat firm."

[1] Referring to Vishnu and Rāma respectively.

Then, if the devotional aspirant is sincere, out of this little seed will come a gigantic tree, like the Indian banyan, sending out branch after branch and root after root to all sides, till it covers the entire field of religion. Thus will the true devotee realize that He who was his own ideal in life is worshipped in all ideals, by all sects, under all names, and through all forms.

HOW TO CULTIVATE BHAKTI

WITH REGARD to the method and the means of bhakti-yoga we read in the commentary of Bhagavān Rāmānuja on the *Vedānta Sutras:* "The attaining of bhakti comes through discrimination, controlling the passions, practice, sacrificial work, purity, strength, and suppression of excessive joy." Viveka, or discrimination, is, according to Rāmānuja, discriminating, among other things, pure food from impure. According to him, food becomes impure for three reasons: (1) from the nature of the food itself, as with garlic and so forth, (2) from its coming from wicked and accursed persons, and (3) from physical impurities, such as dirt or hair and the like. Śruti says: "When the food is pure the sattva element gets purified and the memory becomes unwavering"; and Rāmānuja quotes this from the *Chāndogya Upanishad.*

The question of food has always been one of the most vital questions with the bhaktas. Apart from the extravagance into which some of the bhakti sects have run, there is a great truth underlying this question of food. We must remember that, according to the Sāmkhya philosophy, sattva, rajas, and tamas, which in the state of equilibrium form the undifferentiated prakriti, and in the disturbed condition form the visible universe, are both the substance and the qualities of prakriti. As such they are the materials out of which every human form has been manufactured. And the predominance of sattva material is what is absolutely necessary for spiritual development. The materials which we receive through food into our body structure go a great way to determine our mental constitution; therefore the food we eat has to be particularly taken care of. In this matter as in others, however, the fanaticism into which the disciples invariably fall is not to be laid at the door of the masters.

And this discrimination of food is, after all, of secondary importance. The very same passage quoted above is explained by Śankara in his Bhāshya on the Upanishad in a different way, by giving an entirely different meaning to the word *āhāra*, generally translated as "food." According to him: "That which is gathered in is āhāra. The knowledge of the various sensations, such as sound and the rest, is gathered in for the enjoyment of the embodied self; the purification of this knowledge received through sense perception is called the purification of the food (āhāra). The purification of the food means the acquiring of the knowledge of sensations untouched by the defects of attachment, aversion, and delusion. Therefore such knowledge, or āhāra, being purified, the sattva material of its possessor—the internal organ—will become purified, and the sattva being purified, an unbroken memory of the Infinite One, who has been known in His real nature from the scriptures, will result."

These two explanations are apparently conflicting; yet both are true and necessary. The manipulating and controlling of what may be called the finer body, that is to say, the mind, are no doubt higher functions than the controlling of the grosser body of flesh. But the control of the grosser is absolutely necessary to enable one to arrive at the control of the finer. The beginner, therefore, must pay particular attention to all such dietetic rules as have come down from the line of the accredited teachers. But the extravagant, meaningless fanaticism which has driven religion entirely to the kitchen, as may be noticed in many of our sects—without any hope that the noble truth of that religion will ever come out into the sunlight of spirituality—is a peculiar sort of pure and simple materialism. It is neither jñāna nor bhakti nor karma; it is a special kind of lunacy, and those who pin their souls to it are more likely to go to lunatic asylums than to Brahmaloka. So it stands to reason that discrimination in the choice of food is necessary for the attainment of this higher state of mind, which cannot be easily obtained otherwise.

Controlling the passions is the next thing to be attended to. To restrain the indriyas, or organs, from going towards the objects of the senses, to control them and bring them under the guidance of the will, is the very central virtue in religious culture. Then comes the practice of self-restraint and self-denial. The immense possibilities of divine realization in the soul cannot become actualized without struggle and without such practice on the part of the aspiring devotee. "The mind must always think of the Lord." It is very hard at first to compel the mind to think of the Lord always; but with every new effort the power to do so grows stronger in us. "By practice, O son of Kunti, and by non-attachment is yoga attained," says Śri Krishna in the Gitā. And then as to sacrificial work, it is understood that the "five great sacrifices"[1] have to be performed as usual.

Purity is absolutely the basic discipline, the bedrock upon which the building of bhakti rests. Cleansing the external body and discriminating about food are both easy, but without internal cleanliness and purity these external observances are of no value whatsoever. In the list of the qualities conducive to purity, as given by Rāmānuja, there are enumerated satya, truthfulness; ārjava, sincerity; dayā, doing good to others without any gain to oneself; ahimsā, not injuring others by thought, word, or deed; anabhidhyā, not coveting others' goods, not thinking vain thoughts, and not brooding over injuries received from another.

In this list, the one idea that deserves special notice is ahimsā, non-injury to others. This duty of non-injury is, so to say, obligatory on us in relation to all beings.

---

[1] Every householder commits inevitably the fivefold sin of killing, which results from the use of the pestle and mortar, the grinding-stone, the oven, the water-jar, and the broom. He is absolved from this sin by the performance of the five obligatory duties known as yajna, or sacrifice. The five sacrifices are: devayajna (the offering of sacrifices to the gods), brahmayajna (the teaching and reciting of the scriptures), pitriyajna (the offering of libations of water to the ancestors), nriyajna (the feeding of the hungry), and bhutayajna (the feeding of the lower animals). The performance of these five daily sacrifices, or duties, spiritualizes life and establishes concord and harmony between the living and the dead, as well as between the superhuman, human, and subhuman worlds. The selfish life is transformed into an unselfish one. The individual becomes aware of the interdependence of all beings.

It does not simply mean, as with some, the non-injuring of human beings and mercilessness towards the lower animals; nor does it mean, as with some others, the protecting of cats and dogs and the feeding of ants with sugar, with liberty to injure brother man in every possible way. It is remarkable that almost every good idea in this world can be carried to a disgusting extreme. A good practice carried to an extreme and worked out according to the letter of the law becomes a positive evil. The stinking monks of certain religious sects, who do not bathe lest the vermin on their bodies should be killed, never think of the discomfort and disease they bring to their fellow human beings. They do not, however, belong to the religion of the Vedas.

The test of ahimsā is absence of jealousy. Any man may do a good deed, or make a good gift on the spur of the moment or under the pressure of some superstition or priestcraft; but the real lover of mankind is he who is jealous of none. The so-called great men of the world are seen to become jealous of each other for a small name, for a little fame, and for a few bits of gold. So long as this jealousy exists in a heart, it is far away from the perfection of ahimsā. The cow does not eat meat, nor does the sheep. Are they great yogis, great non-injurers? Any fool may abstain from eating this or that; surely that gives him no more distinction than the herbivorous animals. The man who will mercilessly cheat widows and orphans, and do the vilest deeds for money, is worse than any brute, even if he lives entirely on grass. The man whose heart never cherishes even the thought of injury to anyone, who rejoices at the prosperity of even his greatest enemy

—that man is a bhakta, he is a yogi, he is the guru of all, even though he lives every day of his life on the flesh of swine.

Therefore we must always remember that external practices have value only as they help to develop internal purity. It is better to have internal purity alone, when minute attention to external observances is not practicable. But woe unto the man and woe unto the nation that forgets the real, internal, spiritual essentials of religion and mechanically clutches with death-like grasp all external forms and never lets them go! The forms have value only so far as they are the expressions of the life within. If they have ceased to express life, crush them out without mercy.

The next means to the attainment of bhakti is strength, or anavasāda. "This Ātman is not to be attained by the weak," says Śruti. Both physical weakness and mental weakness are meant here. "The strong, the hardy," are the only fit students. What can puny little decrepit things do? They will break to pieces whenever the mysterious forces of the body and mind are even slightly awakened by the practice of any of the yogas. It is "the young, the healthy, the strong," that can score success. Physical strength, therefore, is absolutely necessary. It is the strong body alone that can bear the shock of the reaction resulting from the attempt to control the organs. He who wants to become a bhakta must be strong, must be healthy. When the miserably weak attempt any of the yogas, they are likely to get some incurable malady or weaken their minds. Voluntarily weakening the body is really no prescription for spiritual enlightenment.

The mentally weak also cannot succeed in attaining Ātman. The person who aspires to be a bhakta must be cheerful. In the Western world the idea of a religious man is that he never smiles, that a dark cloud must always hang over his face, which, again, must be long-drawn, with the jaws almost collapsed. People with emaciated bodies and long faces are fit subjects for the physician; they are not yogis. It is the cheerful mind that can persevere. It is the strong mind that hews its way through a thousand difficulties. And this, the hardest task of all, the cutting of our way out of the net of māyā, is the work reserved only for giant wills.

Yet at the same time excessive mirth, or anuddharsha, should be avoided. Excessive mirth makes us unfit for serious thought. It also fritters away the energies of the mind in vain. The stronger the will, the less the yielding to the sway of the emotions. Excessive hilarity is quite as objectionable as too much of sad seriousness. Religious realization is possible only when the mind is in a steady, peaceful condition of harmonious equilibrium.

It is thus that one may begin to learn how to love the Lord.

THE PREPARATORY RENUNCIATION

WE HAVE FINISHED the consideration of what may be called the preparatory bhakti and shall now enter on the study of parā-bhakti, or supreme devotion. We have to speak of the preparations for the practice of this parā-bhakti. All such preparations are intended only for the purification of the soul. The repetition of names, the rituals, the forms, and the symbols—all these various things are for the purification of the soul.

The greatest purifier among all such things, a purifier without which no one can enter the regions of the higher devotion, is renunciation. This frightens many; yet without it there cannot be any spiritual growth. In all the yogas renunciation is necessary. This is the stepping-stone and the real centre, the real heart, of all spiritual culture—renunciation. This is religion—renunciation. When the human soul draws back from the things of the world and tries to go into deeper things; when man, the Spirit, which has here somehow become concretized and materialized, understands that he is going to be destroyed and reduced almost to mere matter, and turns his face away from matter—then begins renunciation, then begins real spiritual growth.

The karma-yogi's renunciation takes the shape of giving up all the fruits of his actions. He is not attached to the results of his labours; he does not care for any reward here or hereafter. The rāja-yogi knows that the whole of nature is intended as a means for the soul to acquire experience, and that the result of all the experiences of the soul is that it becomes aware of its eternal separateness from nature. The human soul has to understand and realize that it has been Spirit, and not matter, through eternity, and that this conjunction of it with matter is and can be only for a time. The rāja-yogi learns the lesson of renunciation through his own experience of nature. The jnāna-yogi has the harshest of all renunciations to go through, for he has to realize from the very first that the whole of this solid-looking nature is an illusion. He has to understand that any kind of manifestation of power in external nature belongs to the soul and not to nature. He has to know, from the very start, that all knowledge and all experience are in the soul and not in nature; so he has at once and by the sheer force of rational conviction to tear himself away from all bondage to nature. He lets nature and all that belongs to it go; he lets them vanish and tries to stand alone.

Of all renunciations, the most natural, so to say, is that of the bhakti-yogi. Here there is no violence, nothing to give up, nothing to tear off, as it were, from ourselves, nothing from which we have to separate ourselves violently. The bhakta's renunciation is easy, smooth-flowing, and as natural as the things around us. We see the manifestation of this sort of renunciation, although more or less in the form of caricatures, every day around us. A man begins to love a woman; after a while he loves another, and he lets the first woman go. She drops out of his mind smoothly, gently, without his feeling the want of her at all. A woman loves a man; she then begins to love another man, and the first one drops out of her mind quite naturally. A man loves his own city; then he begins to love his country, and the intense love for his little city drops off smoothly, naturally. Again, a man learns to love the whole world; his love for his country, his intense, fanatical patriotism, drops off without hurting him, without any manifestation of violence. An uncultured man loves the pleasures of the senses intensely; as he becomes cultured, he begins to love intellectual pleasures, and his sense enjoyments become less and less intense. No man can enjoy a meal with the same gusto or pleasure as does a dog or a wolf; but those pleasures which a man gets from intellectual experiences and achievements, the dog can never enjoy.

At first, pleasure is associated with the lower sense-organs; but as soon as an animal reaches a higher plane of existence, the lower pleasure becomes less intense. In human society, the nearer a man is to the animal, the stronger is his pleasure in the senses; and the higher and the more cultured a man is, the greater is his pleasure in intellectual and other such finer pursuits. So, when a man goes even higher than the plane of the intellect, higher than that of mere thought, when he reaches the plane of spirituality and of divine inspiration, he finds there a state of bliss compared with which all the pleasures of the senses, or even of the intellect, are as nothing. When the moon shines brightly all the stars become dim, and when the sun shines the moon itself becomes dim. The renunciation necessary for the attainment of bhakti is not obtained by killing anything; it comes naturally, just as, in the presence of an increasingly stronger light, less intense lights become dimmer and dimmer until they vanish away completely.

So this love of the pleasures of the senses and of the intellect is all made dim and thrown aside and cast into the shade by the love of God Himself. That love of God grows and assumes a form called parā-bhakti, or supreme devotion. Forms vanish, rituals fly away, books are superseded; images, temples, churches, religions and sects, countries and nationalities—all these little limitations and bondages fall away naturally from him who knows this love of God. Nothing re-mains to bind him or fetter his freedom. A ship all of a sudden comes near a magnetic rock, and its iron bolts and bars are all attracted and drawn out, and the planks are loosened and float freely on the water. Divine grace thus loosens the binding bolts and bars of the soul, and it becomes free. So in this renuncia-tion auxiliary to devotion there is no harshness, no dryness, no struggle, no repression or suppression. The bhakta has not to suppress any single one of his emo-tions; he only strives to intensify them and direct them to God.

THE BHAKTA'S RENUNCIATION RESULTS FROM LOVE

WE SEE LOVE everywhere in nature. Whatever in society is good and great and sublime is the working out of that love; whatever in society is very bad, nay, diabolical, is also the ill-directed working out of the same emotion of love. It is this same emotion that gives us not only the pure and holy conjugal love between husband and wife, but also the sort of love which goes to satisfy the lowest forms of animal passion. The emotion is the same, but its manifestation is different in different cases. It is the same feeling of love, well or ill directed, that impels one man to do good and to give all he has to the poor, and makes another man cut the throats of his brethren and take away all their possessions. The former loves others as much as the latter loves himself. The direction of the love is bad in the latter case, but is right and proper in the other. The same fire that cooks a meal for us may burn a child, and it is no fault of the fire if it does so; the difference lies in the way in which it is used. Therefore love—the intense longing for association, the strong desire on the part of two to become one, and, it may be after all, of all to become merged in one—is being manifested everywhere in higher or lower forms as the case may be.

Bhakti-yoga is the science of higher love. It shows us how to direct it; it shows us how to control it, how to manage it, how to use it, how to give it a

new aim, as it were, and from it obtain the highest
and most glorious results, that is, how to make it lead
us to spiritual blessedness. Bhakti-yoga does not say,
"Give up"; it only says, "Love—love the Highest."
And everything low naturally falls away from him,
the object of whose love is this Highest.

"I cannot tell anything about Thee except that
Thou art my love. Thou art beautiful—oh, Thou art
beautiful! Thou art beauty itself." What is really
required of us in this yoga is that our thirst after
the beautiful should be directed to God. What is the
beauty in the human face, in the sky, in the stars, and
in the moon? It is only the partial manifestation of the
real, all-embracing Divine Beauty. "He shining, everything shines. It is through His light that all things
shine." Take this high position of bhakti, which makes
you forget at once all your little personalities. Take
yourself away from all the world's little selfish cling-
ings. Do not look upon humanity as the centre of all
your human or higher interests. Stand as a witness,
and observe and study the phenomena of nature. Have
the feeling of non-attachment with regard to man,
and see how this mighty feeling of love is working
itself out in the world. Sometimes a little friction is
produced, but that is only in the course of the struggle to attain the higher, real love. Sometimes there
is a little fight or a little fall; but it is all only by the
way. Stand aside and freely let these frictions come.
You feel the frictions only when you are in the current of the world; but when you are outside it, simply
as a witness and as a student, you will be able to see

that there are millions and millions of channels through which God is manifesting Himself as love.

"Wherever there is any bliss, even though it is of the most sensual kind, there is a spark of that Eternal Bliss which is the Lord Himself." Even in the lowest kinds of attraction there is the germ of divine love. One of the names of the Lord, in Sanskrit, is Hari, and this means "He who attracts all things to Himself." His is in fact the only attraction felt by human hearts. Who can really attract a soul? Only He. Do you think dead matter can truly attract the soul? It never did and never will. When you see a man going after a beautiful face, do you think it is the handful of arranged material molecules which really attracts the man? Not at all. Behind those material particles there must be and is the play of divine influence and divine love. The ignorant man does not know it; but yet, consciously or unconsciously, he is attracted by it and it alone. So even the lowest forms of attraction derive their power from God Himself. "None, O beloved, ever loves the husband for the husband's sake; it is the Ātman, the Lord who is within, for whose sake the husband is loved." Loving wives may know this or they may not; it is true all the same. "None, O beloved, ever loves the wife for the wife's sake; but it is the Self in the wife that is loved." Similarly, no one loves a child or anything else in the world except on account of Him who is within. The Lord is the great magnet, and we are all like iron filings; we are being constantly attracted by Him, and all of us are struggling to reach Him. All this struggling of ours in this world is surely not intended for selfish ends.

Fools do not know what they are doing: the goal of their life is, after all, to approach the great magnet. All the tremendous struggling and fighting in life is intended to make us ultimately go to Him and be one with Him.

The bhakti-yogi, however, knows the meaning of life's struggles; he understands them. He has passed through a long series of these struggles and knows what they mean, and earnestly desires to be free from the friction thereof. He wants to avoid the clash and go direct to the centre of all attraction, the great Hari. This is the renunciation of the bhakta. This mighty attraction in the direction of God makes all other attractions vanish for him; this mighty, infinite love of God which enters his heart leaves no place for any other love to live there. How can it be otherwise? Bhakti fills his heart with the divine waters of the Ocean of Love, which is God Himself; there is no place there for little loves. That is to say, the bhakta's renunciation is that vairāgya, or non-attachment for all things that are not God, which results from anurāga, or great attachment to God.

This is the ideal preparation for the attainment of the supreme bhakti. When this renunciation comes, the gate opens for the soul to pass through and reach the lofty regions of supreme devotion, or parā-bhakti. Then it is that we begin to understand what parā-bhakti is; and the man who has entered into the inner shrine of parā-bhakti alone has the right to say that all forms and symbols are useless to him as aids to religious realization. He alone has attained that supreme state of love commonly called the brotherhood of men. The rest only talk. He sees no distinctions; the mighty Ocean of Love has entered into him, and he sees not man in man, but beholds his Beloved everywhere. Through every face shines to him his Hari. The light in the sun or the moon is all His manifestation. Wherever there is beauty or sublimity, to him it is all His. Such bhaktas are still living; the world is never without them. Though bitten by a serpent, they only say that a messenger came to them from their Beloved. Such men alone have the right to talk of universal brotherhood. They feel no resentment; their minds never react in the form of hatred or jealousy. The external, the sensuous, has vanished for them for ever. How can they be angry, when, through their love, they are always able to see the Reality behind the scenes?

THE NATURALNESS OF BHAKTI-YOGA
AND ITS CENTRAL SECRET

"THOSE WHO WITH constant attention always worship You, and those who worship the Undifferentiated, the Absolute—of these which are the greater yogis?" asked Arjuna of Śri Krishna. The answer was: "Those who, concentrating their minds on Me, worship Me with eternal constancy and are endowed with the highest faith—they are My best worshippers, they are the greatest yogis. Those who worship the Absolute, the Indescribable, the Undifferentiated, the Omnipresent, the Unthinkable, the All-comprehending, the Immovable, and the Eternal, by controlling their organs and having the conviction of sameness with regard to all things—they too, being engaged in doing good to all beings, come to Me alone. But for those whose minds have been devoted to the unmanifested Absolute, the difficulty of the struggle along the way is much greater; for it is indeed with great difficulty that the path of the unmanifested Absolute is trodden by any embodied being. Those who, having offered up all their work unto Me, with entire reliance on Me, meditate on Me and worship Me without any attachment to anything else—them I soon lift up from the ocean of ever recurring births and deaths, since their minds are wholly attached to Me."

Jnāna-yoga and bhakti-yoga are both referred to here. Both may be said to have been defined in the above passage. Jnāna-yoga is grand; it is high philosophy;

178

and almost every human being thinks, curiously enough, that he can surely do everything required of him by this philosophy. But it is really very difficult to live truly the life of a jnāni. We are liable to run into great danger in trying to guide our life by jnāna. This world may be said to contain both persons of demoniacal nature, who think that taking care of the body is the be-all and end-all of existence, and persons of godly nature, who realize that the body is simply a means to an end, an instrument intended for the culture of the soul. The Devil can and indeed does quote the scriptures for his own purpose; and thus the way of knowledge appears to offer justification for what the bad man does, as much as it offers inducements for what the good man does. This is the great danger in jnāna-yoga. But bhakti-yoga is natural, sweet, and gentle; the bhakta does not take such high flights as the jnāna-yogi, and therefore he is not liable to have such big falls. Until the bondages of the soul pass away, it cannot of course be free, whatever may be the nature of the path that the religious man takes.

Here is a passage showing how, with regard to one of the blessed gopis, the soul-binding chains of both merit and demerit were broken: "The intense pleasure of meditating on God took away the binding effects of her good deeds. Then her intense misery of soul in not attaining unto Him washed off all her sinful propensities. And then she became free."

In bhakti-yoga the central secret is, therefore, to know that the various passions and feelings and emotions in the human heart are not wrong in themselves; only they have to be carefully controlled and given a

higher and higher direction, until they attain the very
highest condition of excellence. The highest direction
is that which takes us to God; every other direction is
lower. We find that pleasure and pain are very common and oft-recurring feelings in our lives. When a
man feels pain because he has no wealth or some such
worldly thing, he is giving a wrong direction to the
feeling. Still, pain has its uses. Let a man feel pain
because he has not reached the Highest, because he
has not reached God, and that pain will lead to his
salvation. When you become glad that you have a
handful of coins, you give a wrong direction to the
feeling of joy. It should be given a higher direction;
it should be made to serve the highest ideal. Pleasure
in that kind of ideal must surely be our highest joy.
This same thing is true of all our other feelings. The
bhakta says that not one of them is wrong; he takes
hold of them all and points them unfailingly towards
God.

FORMS OF LOVE-MANIFESTATION

HERE ARE SOME of the forms in which love manifests itself. First, reverence. Why do people feel reverence for temples and holy places? Because God is worshipped there and His presence is associated with all such places. Why do people in every country pay reverence to teachers of religion? It is natural for the human heart to do so, because all such teachers preach the Lord. At bottom, reverence grows out of love; none of us can revere one whom we do not love. Then comes priti, or pleasure in God. What an immense pleasure men take in the objects of the senses! They go anywhere, run through any danger, to get the thing which they love, the thing which their senses crave. What is wanted of the bhakta is this very kind of intense love, which has, however, to be directed to God. Then there is the sweetest of pains, viraha, the intense misery due to the absence of the Beloved. When a man feels intense misery because he has not attained to God, has not known that which is the only thing worthy to be known, and becomes in consequence very dissatisfied and almost mad, then there is viraha; and this state of mind makes him feel disturbed in the presence of anything other than the Beloved. In earthly love we see how often this viraha comes. Again, when men are really and intensely in love with women, or women with men, they feel a kind of natural annoyance in the presence of all those whom they do not love. Exactly the same state of impatience with regard

to things that are not loved comes to the mind when
parā-bhakti holds sway over it. Even to talk about
things other than God becomes distasteful then.
"Think of Him, think of Him alone, and give up all
vain words." The bhakta feels friendly towards those
who talk of Him alone; while those who talk of anything else appear to him to be unfriendly.

A still higher stage of love is reached when life is
maintained only for the sake of the one ideal of love,
when life is considered beautiful and worth living only
on account of that love. Without it, life would not
endure even for a moment. Life is sweet because one
thinks of the Beloved. Tadiyatā, "Hisness," comes
when a man becomes perfect according to bhakti—
when he has become blessed, when he has attained
God, when he has touched the feet of God, as it were.
Then his whole nature is purified and completely
changed. All his purpose in life then becomes fulfilled.
Yet many such bhaktas live on solely to worship Him.
That is the bliss, the only pleasure in life, which they
will not give up. "O king, such is the blessed quality
of Hari that even those who have become satisfied
with the Self, all the knots of whose hearts have been
cut asunder, even they love the Lord for love's sake"—
the Lord, "whom all the gods worship, all the lovers
of liberation, and all the knowers of Brahman." Such
is the power of love. When a man has forgotten himself altogether and does not feel that anything belongs
to him, then he acquires the state of tadiyatā. Everything is sacred to him because it belongs to the Beloved. Even with regard to earthly love, the lover
thinks that everything belonging to his beloved is

sacred and very dear to him. He loves even a piece of the cloth belonging to the darling of his heart. In the same way, when a person loves the Lord the whole universe becomes dear to him, because it is all His.

UNIVERSAL LOVE

H OW CAN WE LOVE the vyashti, the particular, without first loving the samashti, the universal? God
is the samashti, the generalized and abstract universal
whole; and the universe that we see is the vyashti, the
particularized entity. To love the visible universe is
possible only by way of loving the samashti, the universal, which is, as it were, the one unity in which are
to be found millions and millions of smaller unities.
The philosophers of India do not stop at particulars;
they cast a hurried glance at the particulars and immediately start to find the generalized forms which
will include all the particulars. The search after the
universal is the one search of Indian philosophy and
religion. The jnāni aims at the wholeness of things,
at that one absolute and generalized Being by knowing
which he knows everything. The bhakta wishes to
realize that one generalized abstract Person, in loving
whom he loves the whole universe. The yogi wishes
to have possession of that one generalized form of
power by controlling which he controls this whole
universe. The Indian mind, throughout its history,
has been directed to this kind of singular search after
the universal in everything—in science, in psychology,
in love, in philosophy. So the conclusion to which the
bhakta comes is that if you go on merely loving one
person after another, you may go on loving them for
an infinite length of time without being in the least
able to love the world as a whole. When at last, how-

ever, one arrives at the central idea that the sum total
of all love is God, that the sum total of the aspirations
of all the souls in the universe, whether they be free
or bound or struggling towards liberation, is God,
then alone does it become possible for one to manifest
universal love.

God is the samashti, and this visible universe is God
differentiated and made manifest. If we love the sum
total, we love everything. Loving the world and doing
good to it will all come easily then. But we have to
obtain this power by loving God first; otherwise it is
no easy matter to do good to the world. "Everything is
His and He is my Lover. I love Him," says the bhakta.
In this way everything becomes sacred to the bhakta,
because all things are His. All are His children, His
body, His manifestation. How then can we hurt anyone? How then can we dislike anyone? With love of
God will come, as a sure effect, love of everyone in
the universe. The nearer we approach God, the more
do we begin to see that all things are in Him.

When the soul succeeds in enjoying the bliss of this
supreme love, it also begins to see Him in everything.
Our heart thus becomes an eternal fountain of love.
And when we reach even higher states of this love, all
the little differences between the things of the world
are entirely lost. A man is seen no more as a man, but
only as God; an animal is seen no more as an animal,
but as God; even the tiger is no more a tiger, but a
manifestation of God. Thus, in this intense state of
bhakti, worship is offered to everyone—to every life
and to every being. "Knowing that Hari, the Lord, is
in every being, the wise have thus to manifest un-

swerving love towards all beings." As a result of this kind of intense, all-absorbing love comes the feeling of perfect self-surrender, the conviction that nothing that happens is against us. Then the loving soul is able to say, if pain comes, "Welcome, pain!" If misery comes, it will say, "Welcome, misery! You are also from the Beloved." If a serpent comes, it will say, "Welcome, serpent!" If death comes, such a bhakta will welcome it with a smile. "Blessed am I that they all come to me," he will say. "They are all welcome." The bhakta in this state of perfect resignation, arising out of intense love of God and of all that are His, ceases to distinguish between pleasure and pain in so far as they affect him. He does not know what it is to complain of pain or misery; and this kind of uncomplaining resignation to the will of God, who is all love, is indeed a worthier acquisition than all the glory of grand and heroic performances.

To the vast majority of mankind the body is everything. The body is all the universe to them; bodily enjoyment is their all in all. This demon of the worship of the body and of the things of the body has entered into us all. We may indulge in tall talk and take very high flights on the wings of thought, but we are like vultures all the same: our minds are directed to the piece of carrion down below. Why should our body be saved, say, from a tiger? Why may we not give it up to the tiger? The tiger will thereby be pleased, and that is not, after all, so very far from self-sacrifice and worship.

Can you reach the realization of such an idea, in which the sense of self is completely lost? It is a dizzy height, the very pinnacle of the religion of love, and few in this world have ever climbed up to it; but until a man reaches that highest point of ever ready and ever willing self-sacrifice, he cannot become a perfect bhakta. We may all manage to maintain our bodies more or less satisfactorily and for longer or shorter intervals of time. Nevertheless our bodies have to go; there is no permanence about them. Blessed are they whose bodies are destroyed in the service of others. "Wealth, and even life itself, the sage always holds ready for the service of others. In this world, there being one thing certain, namely, death, it is far better that this body die in a good cause than in a bad one." We may drag our life on for fifty years or a hundred years; but after that, what is it that happens? Everything that ·is the result of combination must be dissolved and die. There must and will come a time for it to be decomposed. Jesus and Buddha and Mohammed are all dead; all the great prophets and teachers of the world are dead. "In this evanescent world, where everything is falling to pieces, we have to make the highest use of what we have," says the bhakta; and really the highest use of life is to hold it at the service of all beings.

It is the horrible idea of the body that breeds all the selfishness in the world—just this one delusion that we are wholly the body we own, and that we must by all possible means try our very best to preserve and to please it. If you know that you are positively other than your body, you have then none to fight with or struggle against; you are dead to all ideas of selfishness. So the bhakta declares that we have to hold ourselves as if we are altogether dead to all the things of the world; and that is indeed self-surrender. Let things come as they may. This is the meaning of "Thy will be done"—not going about fighting and struggling, and thinking all the while that God wills all our own weaknesses and worldly ambitions. It may be that good comes even out of our selfish struggles; that is, however, God's look-out. The perfected bhakta's idea must be never to will and work for himself. "Lord, they build high temples in Your name; they make large gifts in Your name. I am poor; I have nothing. So I take this body of mine and place it at Your feet. Do not give me up, O Lord"—such is the prayer proceeding out of the depths of the bhakta's heart.

To him who has experienced it, this eternal sacrifice of the self unto the beloved Lord is higher by far than all wealth and power, even than all soaring thoughts of renown and enjoyment. The peace of the bhakta's calm resignation is a peace that passeth all understanding and is of incomparable value. His self-surrender is a state of the mind in which it has no selfish interests and naturally knows nothing that is opposed to it. In this state of sublime resignation everything in the shape of attachment goes away, except that one all-absorbing love for Him in whom all things live and move and have their being. This attachment of love for God is, indeed, one that does not bind the soul but effectively breaks all its bondages.

THE ONENESS OF THE HIGHER
KNOWLEDGE AND THE HIGHER LOVE

THE UPANISHADS distinguish between a higher knowledge and a lower knowledge; and to the bhakta there is really no difference between this higher knowledge and his higher love, or parā-bhakti. The *Mundaka Upanishad* says: "The knowers of Brahman declare that there are two kinds of knowledge worthy to be known, namely, the higher (parā) and the lower (aparā). Of these, the lower knowledge consists of the Rig-Veda, the Yajur-Veda, the Sāma-Veda, the Atharva-Veda, śikshā (the science dealing with pronunciation and accent), kalpa (the sacrificial liturgy), grammar, nirukta (the science dealing with etymology and the meaning of words), prosody, and astronomy; and the higher knowledge is that by which the Unchangeable is known." The higher knowledge is thus clearly shown to be the Knowledge of Brahman. The *Devi-Bhāgavata* gives us the following definition of the higher love (parā-bhakti): "As oil poured from one vessel to another falls in an unbroken line, so, when the mind in an unbroken stream thinks of the Lord, we have what is called parā-bhakti, or supreme love." This kind of undisturbed and ever steady direction of the mind and heart to the Lord, with an inseparable attachment, is indeed the highest manifestation of man's love for God. All other forms of bhakti are only preparatory to the attainment of this highest form thereof, namely, parā-bhakti, which is also known

189

as rāgānugā, the love that comes after attachment.
When this supreme love once comes into a man's heart,
his mind will continuously think of God and remember nothing else. He will give no room to thoughts
other than those of God; his soul will be unconquer-
ably pure and will break all the bonds of mind and
matter and become serenely free. He alone can worship
the Lord in his own heart; to him forms, symbols,
books, and doctrines are all unnecessary and are incapable of proving serviceable in any way.

It is not easy to love the Lord thus. Ordinarily human love is seen to flourish only in places where it is
returned. Where love is not returned for love, cold
indifference is the natural result. There are, however,
rare instances in which we may notice love exhibiting
itself even where there is no return of love. We may
compare this kind of love, for purposes of illustration,
to the love of the moth for the fire: the insect loves
the fire, falls into it, and dies. It is indeed in the nature
of this insect to love so. To love because it is the nature
of love to love is undeniably the highest and the most
unselfish manifestation of love that can be seen in
the world. Such love working itself out on the plane
of spirituality necessarily leads to the attainment of
parā-bhakti.

THE TRIANGLE OF LOVE

WE MAY REPRESENT love as a triangle, each of the angles of which corresponds to one of its inseparable characteristics. There can be no triangle without its three angles, and there can be no true love without its three following characteristics. The first angle of our triangle of love is that love knows no bargaining. Wherever there is any seeking for something in return, there cannot be any real love; it becomes a mere matter of shopkeeping. So long as there is in us any idea of deriving this or that favour from God in return for our respect and allegiance to Him, there can be no true love growing in our hearts. Those who worship God because they wish Him to bestow favours on them are sure not to worship Him if those favours are not forthcoming. The bhakta loves the Lord because He is lovable; there is no other motive originating or directing this divine emotion of the true devotee.

We have heard it said that a great king once went into a forest and there met a sage. He talked with the sage a little and was very much pleased with his purity and wisdom. The king then wanted the sage to oblige him by receiving a present from him. The sage refused to do so, saying: "The fruits of the forest are enough food for me; the pure streams of water flowing down from the mountains give enough of drink for me; the bark of the trees supplies me with enough of covering; and a cave in the mountains forms my home. Why

should I take any present from you or from anybody?"
The king said, "Just to benefit me, sir, please take
something from my hands and please come with me
to the city and to my palace." After much persuasion
the sage at last consented to do as the king desired,
and went with him to his palace. Before offering the
gift to the sage the king prayed to God repeatedly:
"Lord, give me more children. Lord, give me more
wealth. Lord, give me more territory. Lord, keep my
body in better health"—and so on. Before the king
finished saying his prayers the sage got up and quietly
walked out of the room. On seeing this the king became perplexed and began to follow him, crying aloud:
"Sir, you are going away! You have not received my
gifts." The sage turned round and said to him: "I do
not beg of beggars. You are yourself nothing but a
beggar; and how can you give me anything? I am no
fool to think of taking anything from a beggar like
you. Go away. Do not follow me."

In this story is well brought out the distinction
between mere beggars and the real lovers of God.
Begging is not the language of love. To worship God
even for the sake of salvation or any other reward is
equally degenerate. Love knows no reward. Love is
always for love's sake. The bhakta loves because he
cannot help loving. When you see some beautiful
scenery and fall in love with it, you do not demand
anything in the way of a favour from the scenery;
nor does the scenery demand anything from you. Yet
the vision of it brings you to a blissful state of mind:
it tones down all the friction in your soul; it makes you
calm, almost raises you, for the time being, beyond your

mortal nature, and places you in a condition approaching divine ecstasy. This nature of real love is the first
angle of our triangle. Ask not anything in return for
your love; let your position be always that of the giver.
Give your love unto God, but do not ask anything in
return from Him.

The second angle of the triangle of love is that love
knows no fear. Those who love God through fear are
the lowest of devotees—not fully developed men. They
worship God from fear of punishment. To them He
is a great Being with a whip in one hand and a sceptre
in the other. They are afraid that if they do not obey
Him they will be whipped. It is a degradation to worship God through fear of punishment; such worship
is, if worship at all, the crudest form of worship
through love. So long as there is any fear in the heart,
how can there be love also? Love conquers all fear
naturally. Think of a young mother in the street, and
a dog barking at her; she is frightened and flies into
the nearest house. But suppose the next day she is in
the street with her child, and a lion springs upon the
child. Where will she be now? Of course, in the very
mouth of the lion, protecting her child. Love conquers
all fear. Fear comes from the selfish idea of cutting
oneself off from the universe. The smaller and the
more selfish I make myself, the greater is my fear. If
a man thinks he is a mere nothing, fear will surely
come upon him. And the less you think of yourself
as an insignificant person, the less fear will there be
for you. So long as there is the least spark of fear in
you there can be no love. Love and fear are incom-
patible; God is never to be feared by those who love

Him. The commandment, "Do not take the name of the Lord thy God in vain," the true lover of God laughs at. How can there be any blasphemy in the religion of love? The more you take the name of the Lord, the better for you, in whatever way you may do it. You are only repeating His name because you love Him.

The third angle of the triangle of love is that love knows no rival, for in it is always embodied the lover's highest ideal. True love never comes until the object of our love becomes to us our highest ideal. It may be that in many cases human love is misdirected and misplaced; but to the person who loves, the thing he loves is always his highest ideal. One man may see his ideal in the vilest of beings, and another in the highest of beings; nevertheless in every case it is the ideal alone that is truly and intensely loved. The highest ideal of every man is called God. Ignorant or wise, saint or sinner, man or woman, educated or uneducated, cultivated or uncultivated—to every human being the highest ideal is God. The synthesis of all the highest ideals of beauty, of sublimity, and of power gives us the completest conception of the loving and lovable God. These ideals exist naturally, in some shape or other, in every mind; they form part and parcel of all our minds. All the active manifestations of human nature are struggles of those ideals to become realized in practical life. All the various movements that we see around us in society are caused by the various ideals, in various souls, trying to come out and become concretized; what is inside presses on to come outside. This perennially dominant influence of the ideal is the one force, the one motive power, that may be seen to be constantly working in the midst of mankind.

It may be after hundreds of births, after struggling through thousands of years, that a man finds it is vain to try to make the inner ideal completely mould external conditions and square well with them. After realizing this he no longer tries to project his own ideal on the outside world, but worships the ideal itself as ideal, from the highest standpoint of love. This ideally perfect ideal embraces all lower ideals. Everyone admits the truth of the saying that a lover sees Helen's beauty on an Ethiop's brow. The man who is standing aside as a looker-on sees that love is here misplaced; but the lover sees his Helen all the same, and does not see the Ethiop at all. Helen or Ethiop, the objects of our love are really the centres round which our ideals become crystallized. What is it that the world commonly worships? Certainly not the all-embracing, ideally perfect ideal of the supreme devotee and lover. That ideal which men and women commonly worship is what is in themselves; every person projects his or her own ideal on the outside world and kneels before it. That is why we find that men who are cruel and bloodthirsty conceive of a bloodthirsty God, because they can love only their own highest ideal. That is why good men have a very high ideal of God, and why their ideal is indeed so very different from that of others.

THE GOD OF LOVE IS HIS OWN PROOF

WHAT IS THE IDEAL of the lover who has quite passed beyond the idea of selfishness, of bartering and bargaining, and who knows no fear? Even to the great God such a man will say: "I will give You my all, and I do not want anything from You. Indeed there is nothing I can call my own." When a man has acquired this conviction, his ideal becomes one of perfect love, one of perfect fearlessness born of love. The highest ideal of such a person has no narrowness of particularity about it; it is love universal, love without limits and bonds, love itself, absolute love. This grand ideal of the religion of love is worshipped and loved absolutely as such without the aid of any symbols or suggestions. This is the highest form of parā-bhakti, the worship of such an all-comprehending ideal as the ideal; all the other forms of bhakti are only stages on the way to reach it. All our failures and all our successes in following the religion of love are on the road to the realization of that one ideal. Object after object is taken up, and the inner ideal is successively projected on them all; and all such external objects are found inadequate as expressions of the ever expanding inner ideal and are naturally rejected one after another. At last the aspirant begins to think that it is vain to try to realize the ideal in external objects—that all external objects are as nothing when compared to the ideal itself. And in the course of time he acquires the power of realizing the highest and most generalized abstract ideal entirely as an abstraction that is to him quite alive and real.

When the devotee has reached this point, he is no longer impelled to ask whether God can be demonstrated or not, whether He is omnipotent and omniscient or not. To him He is only the God of Love. He is the highest ideal of love, and that is sufficient for all his purposes. He, as love, is self-evident; it requires no proofs to demonstrate the existence of the beloved to the lover. The magistrate-Gods of other forms of religion may require a good deal of proof to prove them; but the bhakta does not and cannot think of such Gods at all. To him God exists entirely as love. "None, O beloved, loves the husband for the husband's sake; it is for the sake of the Self who is in the husband that the husband is loved. None, O beloved, loves the wife for the wife's sake; it is for the sake of the Self who is in the wife that the wife is loved."

It is said by some that selfishness is the only motive power behind all human activities. That also is love, though it has been lowered by being particularized. When I think of myself as comprehending the Universal, there can surely be no selfishness in me; but when, by mistake, I think that I am something little, my love becomes particularized and narrowed. The mistake consists in making the sphere of love narrow and contracted. All things in the universe are of divine origin and deserve to be loved. It has to be borne in mind, however, that the love of the whole includes the love of the parts.

This whole is the God of the bhaktas; and all the other Gods, Fathers in Heaven, Rulers, or Creators, and all theories and doctrines and books, have no purpose and no meaning for them, seeing that they have through their supreme love and devotion risen above those things altogether. When the heart is purified and cleansed and filled to the brim with the divine nectar of love, all other ideas of God become simply puerile and are rejected as being inadequate or unworthy. Such is indeed the power of parā-bhakti, or supreme love. The perfected bhakta no longer goes to see God in temples and churches; he knows no place where he will not find Him. He finds Him outside the temple as well as in the temple. He finds Him in the wicked man's wickedness as well as in the saint's saintliness, because he has Him already seated in glory in his own heart, as the one almighty, inextinguishable light of love, which is ever shining and eternally present.

HUMAN REPRESENTATIONS OF
DIVINE LOVE

IT IS IMPOSSIBLE to express the nature of this supreme and absolute ideal of love in human language. Even the highest flight of human imagination is incapable of comprehending it in all its infinite perfection and beauty. Nevertheless the followers of the religion of love in its higher as well as its lower forms, in all countries, have all along had to use inadequate human language to comprehend and to define their own ideal of love. Nay, human love itself, in all its varied forms, has been made to typify this inexpressible divine love. Man can think of divine things only in his own human way; to us the Absolute can be expressed only in our relative language. The whole universe is to us a writing of the Infinite in the language of the finite. Therefore bhaktas make use, in relation to God and His worship through love, of all the common terms associated with the common love of humanity.

Some of the great writers on parā-bhakti have tried to understand and experience this divine love in a number of different ways. The lowest form in which this love is apprehended is what they call the peaceful, the śānta. When a man worships God without the fire of love in him, without its madness in his brain, when his love is just the calm, commonplace love, a little higher than mere forms and ceremonies and symbols, but not at all characterized by the madness of intensely active love, it is said to be śānta. We see some people

in the world who like to move on slowly, and others
who come and go like the whirlwind. The śānta-
bhakta is calm, peaceful, gentle.

The next higher type is that of dāsya, servantship.
It comes when a man thinks he is the servant of the
Lord. The attachment of the faithful servant to the
master is his ideal.

The next type of love is sakhya, friendship—"Thou
art our beloved friend." Just as a man opens his heart
to his friend and knows that the friend will never
chide him for his faults, but will always try to help
him; just as there is the idea of equality between him
and his friend—so equal love flows in and out between
the worshipper and his friendly God. Thus God becomes our friend, the friend who is near, the friend to
whom we may freely tell all the tales of our lives,
before whom we may place the innermost secrets of
our hearts with the greatest assurance of safety and
support. He is the friend whom the devotee accepts as
an equal. God is viewed here as our playmate.

We may well say that we are all playing in this
universe. Just as children play their games, just as
the most glorious kings and emperors play their own
games, so is the beloved Lord Himself playing in this
universe. He is perfect. He does not want anything.
Why should He create? Activity, with us, is always
for the fulfilment of a certain want; and want always
presupposes imperfection. God is perfect. He has no
wants. Why should He go on with this incessant work
of creation? What purpose could He have in view?
The stories of God's creating the world for some end
or other that we imagine, are good as stories, but not

otherwise. It is all really sport; the universe is merely His play. The whole universe must after all be a big piece of pleasing fun to Him. If you are poor enjoy being poor, as fun; if you are rich enjoy the fun of being rich; if dangers come it is also good fun; if happiness comes there is more good fun. The world is just a playground, and we are here having good fun, having a game; and God is playing with us all the while, and we are playing with Him. God is our eternal playmate. How beautifully He is playing! The play is finished when the cycle comes to an end. There is rest for a shorter or longer time; again all come out and play.

It is only when you forget that it is all play and that you are also helping in the play—it is only then that misery and sorrows come, that the heart becomes heavy, that the world weighs upon you with tremendous power. But as soon as you give up your serious belief in the reality of the changing incidents of the three minutes of life, and know it to be but a stage on which you are playing, helping Him to play, at once misery ceases for you. He plays in every atom. He is playing when He is building up earths and suns and moons. He is playing with the human heart, with animals, with plants. We are His chessmen: He puts the chessmen on the board and shakes them up. He arranges us first in one way and then in another, and we consciously or unconsciously help in His play. And oh, bliss! we are His playmates.

The next type of love is what is known as vātsalya, loving God not as our father but as our child. This may seem peculiar, but it is a discipline to enable us to detach all ideas of power from the concept of God. The idea of power brings with it awe. There should be no awe in love. The ideas of reverence and obedience are necessary for the formation of character; but when character is formed, when the lover has tasted the calm peaceful love and tasted also a little of love's intense madness, then he need talk no more of ethics and discipline. The lover says he does not care to conceive of God as mighty, majestic, and glorious, as the Lord of the universe or as the God of gods. It is to avoid this association with God of the fear-creating sense of power that he worships God as his own child. The mother and the father are not moved by awe in relation to the child. They cannot have any reverence for the child. They cannot think of asking any favour of him. The child's position is always that of the receiver; and out of love for him the parents will give up their bodies a hundred times over. A thousand lives they will sacrifice for that one child of theirs. And therefore God is loved as a child.

This idea of loving God as a child comes into existence and grows naturally among those religious sects which believe in the incarnation of God. For the Mohammedans it is impossible to have this idea of God as a child; they would shrink from it with a kind of horror. But the Christians and the Hindus can realize it easily, because they have the Baby Jesus and the Baby Krishna. The women in India often look upon themselves as Krishna's mother. Christian mothers also may take up the idea that they are Christ's mother; and it will bring to the West the knowledge of God's divine Motherhood, which they so much need. The superstitions of awe and reverence in relation to God are deeply rooted in our heart of hearts, and it takes long years to sink entirely in love our ideas of reverence and veneration, of awe and majesty and glory, with regard to God.

There is one more human representation of the divine ideal of love. It is known as the madhura, the sweetheart relationship, and is the highest of all such representations. It is indeed based on the highest manifestation of love in this world, and this love is also the strongest known to man. What love shakes the whole nature of man, what love runs through every particle of his being, makes him mad, makes him forget his own nature, transforms him, makes him either a god or a demon, as does the love between man and woman? In this sweet representation of divine love God is our husband. We are all women; there are no men in this world. There is but one Man, and that is He, our Beloved. All that love which man gives to woman, or woman to man, has here to be given to the Lord.

All the different kinds of love which we see in the world, and with which we are more or less merely playing, have God as the one goal. But unfortunately man does not know the infinite Ocean into which this mighty river of love is constantly flowing, and so, foolishly, he often tries to direct it to little dolls of human beings. The tremendous love for the child that is in human nature is not for the little doll of a child. If you bestow it blindly and exclusively on the child, you will suffer in consequence. But through such suffering will come the awakening by which you are sure to find out that the love which is in you, if it is given to any human being, will sooner or later bring pain and sorrow as the result. Our love must therefore be given to the Highest One, who never dies and never changes, to Him in the ocean of whose love there is neither ebb nor flow. Love must reach its right destination; it must go unto Him who is really the infinite Ocean of Love. All rivers flow into the ocean. Even the drop of water coming down from the mountain-side cannot stop its course after reaching a brook or a river, however big; at last even that drop somehow does find its way to the ocean.

God is the one goal of all our passions and emotions. If you want to be angry, be angry with Him. Chide your Beloved; chide your Friend. Whom else can you safely chide? Mortal man will not patiently put up with your anger; there will be a reaction. If you are angry with me, I am sure to react quickly, because I cannot patiently put up with your anger. Say unto the Beloved: "Why do You not come to me? Why do You leave me thus alone?" Where is there any enjoyment but in Him? What enjoyment can there be in little clods of earth? It is the crystallized essence of infinite enjoyment that we have to seek— and that is in God. Let all our passions and emotions go up unto Him. They are meant for Him, for if they miss their mark and go lower, they become vile. When they go straight to the mark, to the Lord, even the lowest of them becomes transfigured; all the energies of the human body and mind, howsoever they may express themselves, have the Lord as their one goal. All loves and all passions of the human heart must go to God. He is the Beloved. Whom else can this heart love? He is the most beautiful, the most sublime; He is beauty itself, sublimity itself. Who in this universe is more beautiful than he? Who in this universe is more fit to become the husband than He? Who in this universe is more fit to be loved than He? So let Him be the Husband; let Him be the Beloved.

Often it so happens that divine lovers who sing of this divine love accept the language of human love in all its aspects as adequate to describe it. Fools do not understand this; they never will. They look at it only with the physical eye. They do not understand the mad throes of this spiritual love. How can they? "Oh, for one kiss of Thy lips, Beloved! One who has been kissed by Thee—his thirst for Thee increases for ever, all his sorrows vanish, and he forgets all things except Thee alone." Aspire after that kiss of the Beloved, that touch of His lips which makes the bhakta mad, which makes of man a god. To him who has been blessed with such a kiss, the whole of nature changes, worlds vanish, suns and moons die out, and the universe itself melts away into that one infinite Ocean of Love. That is the perfection of the madness of love.

Ay, the true spiritual lover does not rest even there; even the love of husband and wife is not mad enough for him. The bhaktas take up also the idea of illegitimate love, because it is so strong. The impropriety of it is not at all the thing they have in view. The nature of this love is such that the more obstructions there are to its free play, the more passionate it becomes. The love between husband and wife is smooth; there are no obstructions there. So the bhaktas take up the idea of a girl who is in love with a man—and her mother or father or her husband objects to that love, and the more anybody obstructs the course of her love, the more her love tends to grow in strength. Human language cannot describe how madly the ever blessed gopis loved Krishna in the groves of Vrindā, how at the sound of His flute they rushed out to meet Him, forgetting everything, forgetting this world and its ties, its duties, its joys and its sorrows.

Man, O man! you speak of divine love and at the same time are able to attend to all the vanities of this world. Are you sincere? "Where Rāma is, there is no room for any desire; where desire is, there is no room for Rāma. These never co-exist. Like light and darkness they are never together."

CONCLUSION

WHEN THIS HIGHEST IDEAL of love is reached, philosophy is thrown away. Who will then care for it? Freedom, salvation, Nirvāna—all are thrown away. Who cares to become free while in the enjoyment of divine love? "Lord, I do not want wealth, or friends, or beauty, or learning, or even freedom. Let me be born again and again, and be Thou ever my Love. Be Thou ever and ever my Love." "Who cares to become sugar?" says the bhakta. "I want to taste sugar." Who will then desire to become free and one with God? "I may know that I am He; yet I will take myself away from Him and become different, so that I may enjoy the Beloved." That is what the bhakta says. Love for love's sake is his highest enjoyment. Who would not be bound hand and foot a thousand times over to enjoy the Beloved?

No bhakta cares for anything except love—except to love and be loved. His motiveless love is like the tide rushing up the river. The lover goes up the river, against the current. The world calls him mad. I know one whom the world used to call mad, and this was his answer: "My friends, the whole world is a lunatic asylum. Some are mad after worldly love, some after name, some after fame, some after money, some after salvation and going to heaven. In this big lunatic asylum I am also mad—I am mad after God. If you are mad after money, I am mad after God. You are mad; so am I. I think my madness is after all the best."

The true bhakta's love is this burning madness, before which everything else vanishes for him. The whole universe is to him full of love and love alone; that is how it seems to the lover. So when a man has this love in him, he becomes eternally blessed, eternally happy. He has drawn near to God; he has thrown off all those vain desires with which he was filled before. And with his desires, selfishness has vanished. This blessed madness of divine love alone can cure for ever the disease of the world that is in us.

We all have to begin as dualists in the religion of love. God is to us a separate Being, and we feel ourselves to be separate beings also. Love then comes between, and man begins to approach God; and God also comes nearer and nearer to man. Man takes up all the various relationships of life—such as father, mother, son, friend, master, lover—and projects them on his ideal of love, on his God. To him God exists as all these. And the last point of his progress is reached when he feels that he has become absolutely merged in the object of his worship.

We all begin with love for ourselves, and the unfair claims of the little self make even love selfish. At last, however, comes the full blaze of light, in which this little self is seen to have become one with the Infinite. Man himself is transfigured in the presence of this light of love, and he realizes at last the beautiful and inspiring truth that love, the lover, and the Beloved are one.

MISCELLANEOUS
LECTURES

WHAT IS RELIGION?

A HUGE LOCOMOTIVE rushes on down the tracks, and a small worm that has been creeping upon one of the rails saves its life by crawling out of the path of the locomotive. Yet this little worm, so insignificant that it can be crushed in a moment, is a living something, while the locomotive, so huge, so immense, is only an engine, a machine. You see, the one has life and the other is only dead matter, and all its power and strength and speed are only those of a dead machine, a mechanical contrivance. The poor little worm which moves upon the rail and which the least touch of the engine would surely deprive of its life is a majestic being compared to that huge locomotive. It is a small part of the Infinite and therefore it is greater than the powerful engine. Why should that be so? How do we know the living from the dead? The machine mechanically performs all the movements its maker made it to perform; its movements are not those of life. How can we make the distinction between the living and the dead, then? In the living there is freedom, there is intelligence; in the dead all is bound and no freedom is possible, because there is no intelligence. This freedom that distinguishes us from mere machines is what we are all striving for. To be more free is the goal of all our efforts; for only in perfect freedom can there be perfection. This effort to attain freedom underlies all forms of worship, whether we know it or not.

If we were to examine the various sorts of worship all over the world, we would see that the crudest of mankind are worshipping ghosts, demons, and the spirits of their forefathers. Serpent-worship, worship of tribal gods, and worship of the departed ones—why do they practise all this? Because they feel that in some unknown way these beings are greater, more powerful, than themselves and so limit their freedom. They therefore seek to propitiate these beings in order to prevent them from molesting them—in other words, to get more freedom. They also seek to win favour from these superior beings, to get as a gift what ought to be earned by personal effort.

On the whole, this shows that the world is expecting a miracle. This expectation never leaves us, and however we may try, we are all running after the miraculous and extraordinary. What is mind but that ceaseless inquiry into the meaning and mystery of life? We may say that only uncultivated people are going after all these things; but the question still is there— why should it be so? The Jews were asking for a miracle. The whole world has been asking for the same thing these thousands of years.

There is, again, the universal dissatisfaction: we take up an ideal, but we have rushed only half the way after it when we take up a new one. We struggle hard to attain a certain goal and then discover we do not want it. This dissatisfaction we are experiencing time after time; and what is there in life if there is to be only dissatisfaction? What is the meaning of this universal dissatisfaction? It indicates that freedom is every man's goal. He seeks it ever; his whole life is a struggle after it. The child rebels against law as soon as it is born. Its first utterance is a cry, a protest against the bondage in which it finds itself. This longing for freedom produces the idea of a Being who is absolutely free. The concept of God is a fundamental element in the human constitution. Satchidānanda, Existence-Knowledge-Bliss, is, in Vedānta, the highest concept of God possible to the mind. It is by its nature the Essence of Knowledge and the Essence of Bliss. We have been stifling that inner voice, seeking to follow law and suppress our true nature; but there is that human instinct to rebel against nature's laws.

We may not understand what all this means; but there is that unconscious struggle of the human with the spiritual, of the lower with the higher mind, and through this struggle we attempt to preserve our separate life, what we call our "individuality." Even hell illustrates this miraculous fact that we are born rebels. Against the inevitable facts of life we rebel and cry out, "No law for us!" As long as we obey the laws we are like machines; and the universe goes on and we cannot change it. Laws become man's nature. The first inkling of life on its higher level is in seeing this struggle within us to break the bonds of nature and to be free. "Freedom, oh, freedom! Freedom, oh, freedom!" is the song of the soul. Bondage, alas—to be bound in nature—seems its fate.

Why should there be serpent-worship or ghost-worship or demon-worship and all the various creeds and forms for the obtaining of miracles? Why do we say that there is life, there is being, in anything? There must be a meaning in all this search, this endeavour to understand life, to explain being. It is not meaningless and vain. It is man's ceaseless endeavour to become free. The knowledge which we now call science has been struggling for thousands of years in its attempt to gain freedom, and people still ask for freedom. Yet there is no freedom in nature. It is all law. Still the struggle goes on. Nay, the whole of nature, from the very sun down to the atoms, is under law, and even for man there is no freedom. But we cannot believe it. We have been studying laws from the beginning and yet cannot—nay, will not—believe that man is under law. The soul cries ever, "Freedom, oh, freedom!"

With the conception of God as a perfectly free Being, man cannot rest eternally in this bondage. Higher he must go, and were the struggle not for freedom he would think it too severe. Man says to himself: "I am a born slave, I am bound; nevertheless there is a Being who is not bound by nature. He is free and the Master of nature." The conception of God, therefore, is as essential and as fundamental a part of the mind as is the idea of bondage. Both are the outcome of the idea of freedom. There cannot be life, even in the plant, without the idea of freedom. In the plant or in the worm, life has to rise to the concept of individuality; it is there, unconsciously working. The plant lives in order to preserve a principle; it is not simply nature. The idea of nature's controlling every step onward overrules the idea of freedom. Onward goes the material world, onward moves the idea of freedom. Still the fight goes on. We are hearing about all the quarrels of creeds and sects;

yet creeds and sects are just and proper; they must be there. They no doubt lengthen the chain, and naturally the struggle increases; but there will be no quarrels if we only know that we are all striving to reach the same goal.

The embodiment of freedom, the Master of nature, is what we call God. You cannot deny Him. No, because you cannot move or live without the idea of freedom. Would you come here if you did not believe you were free? It is quite possible that the biologist can and will give some explanation of this perpetual effort to be free. Taking all that for granted, still the idea of freedom is there. It is a fact, as much so as the other fact that you cannot apparently get over, the fact of being under nature.

Bondage and liberty, light and shadow, good and evil, must be there; but the very fact of the bondage shows also this freedom hidden there. If one is a fact, the other is equally a fact. There must be this idea of freedom. While now we cannot see that this idea of bondage, in uncultivated man, is his struggle for freedom, yet the idea of freedom is there. The consciousness of the bondage of sin and impurity in the uncultivated savage is very slight; for his nature is only a little higher than that of the animal. What he struggles against is the bondage of physical nature, the lack of physical gratification; but out of this lower consciousness grows and broadens the higher conception of a mental or moral bondage and a longing for spiritual freedom. Here we see the divine dimly shining through the veil of ignorance. The veil is very dense at first, and the light may be almost obscured, but it is there, ever pure and undimmed—the radiant light of freedom and perfection. Man personifies this as the Ruler of the universe, the one free Being. He does not yet know that the universe is all one, that the difference is only in the concept and not in things themselves.

The whole of nature is worship of God. Wherever there is life there is this search for freedom, and that freedom is the same as God. Necessarily freedom gives us mastery over all nature and is impossible without knowledge. The more we know, the more we become masters of nature. Mastery alone makes us strong; and if there be some being who is entirely free and a master of nature, that being must have a perfect knowledge of nature, must be omnipresent and om-niscient. Freedom must go hand in hand with these; and only that being who has acquired these will be beyond nature.

Blessedness, eternal peace, arising from perfect free-dom, is the highest concept of religion, underlying all the ideas of God in Vedānta: absolutely free existence, not bound by anything—no change, no nature, noth-ing that can produce a change in Him. This same freedom is in you and in me and is the only real freedom.

God is always established upon His own majestic changeless Self. You and I try to be one with Him, but find ourselves diverted by nature, by the trifles of daily life, by money, by fame, by human love, and all these changing forms which make for bondage. When nature shines, upon what depends its shining? Upon God, and not upon the sun or the moon or the stars.

Wherever anything shines, whether it is the light in the sun or in our own consciousness, it is He. He shining, all shines after Him.

Now, we have seen that this God is self-evident, impersonal, omniscient, the Knower and Master of nature, the Lord of all. He is behind all worship, and all worship is directed to Him whether we know it or not. I go one step farther: That which we call evil is His worship too. This too is a part of freedom. When you are doing evil, the impulse behind is that of freedom. It may be misguided and misled, but it is there, and there cannot be any life or any impulse unless that freedom is behind it. Freedom throbs in the heart of the universe. Such is the conception of the Lord in the Upanishads.

Sometimes it rises even higher, presenting to us an ideal before which at first we stand aghast: that we are in essence one with God. He who is the colouring in the wings of the butterfly and the blossoming of the rose-bud is the power that is in the plant and in the butterfly. He who gives us life is the power within us. Out of His power comes life, and the direst death is also His power. He whose shadow is death—His shadow is immortality also.

Take a still higher conception; see how we are flying like hunted hares from all that is terrible, and like them hiding our heads and thinking we are safe. See how the whole world is flying from everything terrible. Once when I was in Benares, I was passing through a place where there was a large reservoir of water on one side and a high wall on the other. There were many monkeys around that place. The monkeys of Benares are huge brutes and are sometimes surly. They now took it into their heads not to allow me to pass through their street; so they howled and shrieked and clutched at my feet as I passed. As they pressed closer, I began to run; but the faster I ran, the faster came the monkeys, and they began to bite at me. It seemed impossible to escape. But just then I met a stranger, who called out to me, "Face the brutes." I turned and faced the monkeys and they fell back and finally fled. That is a lesson for all life: face the terrible, face it boldly. Like the monkeys, the hardships of life fall back when we cease to flee before them. If we are ever to gain freedom, it must be by conquering nature, never by running away. Cowards never win victories. We have to fight fear and troubles and ignorance if we expect them to flee before us.

What is death? What are terrors? Do you not see the Lord's face in them? Fly from evil and terror and misery and they will follow you. Face them and they will flee. The whole world worships ease and pleasure, and very few dare to worship what is painful. To rise above both is the ideal of freedom. Unless a man passes through pleasure and pain he is not free. We have to face them. We strive to worship the Lord, but the body comes between, nature comes between Him and us and blinds our vision. We must learn how to worship and love Him in the thunderbolt, in shame, in sorrow, in sin. All the world has ever been preaching the God of virtue. I preach a God of virtue and a God of sin in one. Take Him if you dare. That is the one way to salvation. Then alone will come to us the Truth Ultimate which comes from the idea of

Oneness. Then will be lost the idea that one is greater than another. The nearer we approach the ideal of freedom, the more we shall come under the Lord and troubles will vanish. Then we shall not differentiate the door of hell from the gate of heaven, nor differentiate between men and say, "I am greater than any other being in the universe." Until we see nothing in the world but the Lord Himself, all these evils will beset us and we shall make all these distinctions; for it is only in the Lord, in the Spirit, that we are all one, and until we see God everywhere, this unity will not exist for us.

The man who is groping through sin, through misery, the man who is choosing the path through hell, will reach freedom, but it will take time. We cannot help him. Some hard knocks on his head will make him turn to the Lord. The path of virtue, purity, unselfishness, spirituality, he will know at last, and what he has been doing unconsciously he will do consciously. The idea is expressed by St. Paul: "Whom therefore ye ignorantly worship, Him declare I unto you." This is the lesson for the whole world to learn. What have these philosophies and theories of nature to do, if not to help us to attain this one goal in life? Let us come to that consciousness of the identity of everything and let man see himself in everything. Let us be no more the worshippers of creeds or sects with small, limited notions of God, but see Him in everything in the universe. If you are knowers of God, you will everywhere find the same worship as in your own heart.

Get rid, in the first place, of all these limited ideas

and see God in every person—working through all hands, walking through all feet, and eating through every mouth. In every being He lives, through all minds He thinks. He is self-evident, nearer unto us than ourselves. To know this is religion, is faith. May it please the Lord to give us this faith! When we shall feel that Oneness we shall be immortal. We are immortal even physically: one with the universe. So long as there is one that breathes throughout the universe, I live in that one. I am not this limited little being; I am the Universal. I am the life of all the Sons of God. I am the soul of Buddha, of Jesus, of Mohammed. I am the soul of all the teachers, and I am the soul of all the robbers that robbed and of all the murderers that were hanged. Stand up then! This is the highest worship. You are one with the universe. That alone is humility—not crawling upon all fours and calling yourself a sinner. That is the highest evolution when this veil of differentiation is torn off. The highest creed is Oneness. I am So-and-so—is a limited idea, not true of the real "I." I am the Universal: stand upon that and ever worship the Highest through the highest form; for God is Spirit and should be worshipped in Spirit and in Truth. Through lower forms of worship man's materialistic thoughts rise to spiritual worship, and the universal Infinite One is at last worshipped in and through the Spirit. That which is limited is material. The Spirit alone is infinite. God is Spirit, is infinite; man is Spirit and therefore infinite; and the Infinite alone can worship the Infinite. We will worship the Infinite; that is the highest spiritual worship. How grand these ideas are, and how difficult to realize! I theorize, talk, philosophize, and the next moment I come up against something and I unconsciously become angry; I forget there is anything in the universe but this little limited self. I forget to say: "I am the Spirit, what is this trifle to me? I am the Spirit." I forget it is all myself playing. I forget God; I forget freedom.

Sharp as the blade of a razor, long and difficult and hard to cross, is the way to freedom. The sages have declared this again and again. Yet do not let these weaknesses and failures deter you. The Upanishads have declared: "Arise! Awake! and stop not until the goal is reached." We shall then certainly cross the path, sharp as it is, like the razor, and long and distant and difficult though it be. Man becomes the master of gods and demons. No one is to blame for our miseries but ourselves. Do you think there is only a dark cup of poison if man goes to look for nectar? The nectar is there and is for every man who strives to reach it. The Lord Himself tells us: "Give up all these paths and struggles. Do thou take refuge in Me. I will take thee to the other shore; be not afraid." We hear that from all the scriptures of the world that have come to us.

The same voice teaches us to say, "Thy will be done on earth as it is in heaven, for Thine is the kingdom and the power and the glory." It is difficult, all very difficult. I say to myself this moment: "I will take refuge in Thee, O Lord; unto Thy love I will sacrifice all, and on Thine altar I will place all that is good and virtuous. My sins, my sorrows, my actions, good and evil, I will offer unto Thee; do Thou take them and I will never forget." One moment I say, "Thy will be done," and the next moment something comes to try me and I spring up in a rage. The goal of all religions is the same, but the language of the teachers differs. The goal is to kill the false "I" so that the real "I," the Lord, will reign. "I, the Lord, am a jealous God. Thou shalt have no other God but Me," say the Hebrew scriptures. We must cherish God alone. We must say, "Not I, but Thou," and then we should give up everything but the Lord. He, and He alone, should reign. Perhaps we struggle hard and yet the next moment our feet slip, and then we try to stretch out our hands to Mother. We find we cannot stand alone. Life is infinite, one chapter of which is, "Thy will be done," and unless we realize all the chapters we cannot realize the whole.

"Thy will be done"—every moment the traitor mind rebels against it; yet it must be said again and again if we are to conquer the lower self. We cannot serve a traitor and yet be saved. There is salvation for all except the traitor, and we stand condemned as traitors —traitors against our own selves, against the majesty of God—when we refuse to obey the voice of our higher Self. Come what will, we must give our bodies and minds up to the Supreme Will. Well has it been said by the Hindu philosopher, "If man says twice, 'Thy will be done,' he commits sin." "Thy will be done"—what more is needed? Why say it twice? What is good is good. No more shall we take it back. "Thy will be done on earth as it is in heaven, for Thine is the kingdom and the power and the glory for evermore."

BUDDHA'S MESSAGE TO THE WORLD

(Delivered in San Francisco, March 18, 1900)

BUDDHISM IS HISTORICALLY the most important religion—historically, not philosophically—because it was the most tremendous religious movement that the world ever saw, the most gigantic spiritual wave ever to burst upon human society. There is no civilization on which its effect has not been felt in some way or other.

The followers of Buddha were most enthusiastic and very missionary in spirit. They were the first among the adherents of the various religions not to remain content with the limited sphere of their mother church. They spread far and wide; they travelled east and west, north and south. They reached into darkest Tibet; they went into Persia, Asia Minor; they went into Russia, Poland, and many other countries of the Western world. They went into China, Korea, Japan; they went into Burma, Siam, the East Indies, and beyond. When Alexander the Great, through his military conquests, brought the Mediterranean world in contact with India, the wisdom of India at once found a channel through which to spread over vast portions of Asia and Europe. Buddhist priests went out teaching among the different nations, and as they taught, superstition and priestcraft began to vanish like mist before the sun.

To understand this movement properly you should

223

know what conditions prevailed in India when Buddha was born, just as to understand Christianity you have to grasp the state of Jewish society at the time of Christ. It is necessary that you have an idea of Indian society six hundred years before the birth of Christ, by which time Indian civilization had already completed its growth.

When you study the civilization of India you find that it has died and revived several times; this is its peculiarity. Most races rise once and then decline for ever. There are two kinds of peoples: those who grow continually and those whose growth comes to an end. The peaceful nations, India and China, fall down, yet rise again. But the others, once they go down, do not come up; they die. Blessed are the peacemakers, for they shall enjoy the earth.

At the time Buddha was born, India was in need of a great spiritual leader, a prophet. There was already a most powerful body of priests. You will understand the situation better if you remember the history of the Jews—how they had two types of religious leaders: priests and prophets, the priests keeping the people in ignorance and grinding superstitions into their minds. The methods of worship the priests prescribed were only a means by which they could dominate the people. All through the Old Testament you find the prophets challenging the superstitions of the priests. The outcome of this fight was the triumph of the prophets and the defeat of the priests.

Priests believe that there is a God, but that this God can be approached and known only through them. People can enter the holy of holies only with the permission of the priests. You must pay them, worship them, place everything in their hands. Throughout the history of the world this priestly desire for power has asserted itself; this tremendous thirst for power, this tiger-like thirst, seems a part of human nature. The priests dominate you, lay down a thousand rules for you. They describe simple truths in roundabout ways. They tell you stories to support their own superior position. If you want to thrive in this life or go to heaven after death, you have to pass through their hands. You have to perform all kinds of ceremonies and rituals. All this has made life so complicated and has so confused the brain that if I give you plain words you will go home unsatisfied. You have become thoroughly befuddled. The less you understand, the better you feel! The prophets have been giving warnings against the priests and their superstitions and machinations; but the vast mass of people have not yet learnt to heed these warnings; they must be educated about this.

Men must have education. They speak of democracy, of the equality of all men, these days. But how will a man know he is equal with all? He must have a strong brain, a clear mind free of nonsensical ideas; he must pierce through the mass of superstitions encrusting his mind to the pure truth that is in his inmost self. Then he will know that all perfections, all powers, are already within himself; that these have not to be given him by others. The moment he realizes this truth he becomes free, he achieves equality. He also realizes that everyone else is just as perfect as he, and that he does not have to exercise any power—

physical, mental, or moral—over his brother men. He abandons the idea that there was ever any man who was lower than himself. Then he can talk of equality —not until then.

Now, as I was telling you, among the Jews there was a continuous struggle between the priests and the prophets, and the priests sought to monopolize power and knowledge, till they themselves began to lose them and the chains they had put on the feet of the people were on their own feet. The masters always become slaves before long. The culmination of the struggle was the victory of Jesus of Nazareth. This triumph is the history of Christianity; Christ at last succeeded in overthrowing the mass of priestcraft. This great prophet killed the dragon of priestly selfishness, rescued from its clutches the jewel of truth, and gave it to all the world, so that whosoever desired to possess it would have absolute freedom to do so and would not have to wait on the pleasure of any priest or priests.

The Jews were never a very philosophical race; they had not the subtlety of the Indian brain nor did they have the Indian's psychic power. The priests in India, the brāhmins, possessed great intellectual and psychic power. It was they who began the spiritual development of India, and they accomplished wonderful things. But the time came when the free spirit of development that had at first actuated the brāhmins disappeared. They began to arrogate powers and privileges to themselves. If a brāhmin killed a man he would not be punished. The brāhmin, by his very birth, is the lord of the universe. Even the most wicked brāhmin must be worshipped.

But while the priests were flourishing, there existed also the poet-prophets called sannyāsins. All Hindus, whatever their caste may be, must, if they want to attain freedom, give up the world and prepare for death. No more is the world to be of any interest to them. They must go out and become sannyāsins. The sannyāsins have nothing to do with the two thousand ceremonies that the priests have invented—sanctifying them with certain words, ten syllables, twenty syllables long, and so on! All these things are nonsense.

So these poet-prophets of ancient India repudiated the ways of the priests and declared the pure truth. They tried to break the power of the priests and they succeeded a little. But in two generations their disciples went back to the superstitious, roundabout ways of the priests and became priests themselves: "You can get truth only through us." Truth became crystallized again, and again prophets came to break the encrustations and free the truth, and so it went on. Yes, there must always be prophets in the world; otherwise humanity will perish.

You wonder why there have to be all these roundabout methods of the priests. Why can you not come directly to the truth? Are you ashamed of God's truth, that you have to hide it behind all kinds of intricate ceremonies and formulas? Are you ashamed of God, that you cannot confess His truth before the world? Do you call that being religious and spiritual? The priests are the only people fit for the truth! The masses are not fit for it! It must be diluted! Water it down a little!

Take the Sermon on the Mount and the Gitā: they are simplicity itself. Even the man in the street can understand them. How grand! In them you find the truth clearly and simply revealed. But no, the priests will not agree that truth can be found so directly. They speak of two thousand heavens and two thousand hells. If people follow their prescriptions they will go to heaven! If they do not obey the rules they will go to hell!

But people must know the truth. Some are afraid that if the full truth is given to all, it will hurt them. They should not be given the unqualified truth, they say. But the world is not much better off by compromising truth. How much worse can it be than it is already? Bring the truth out! If it is real, it will do good. When people protest and propose other methods, they only make apologies for priestcraft.

India was full of it in Buddha's day. Masses of people were debarred from all knowledge. If just a word of the Vedas entered the ears of a low-caste man, terrible punishment was visited upon him. The priests had made a secret of the Vedas—the Vedas, which contained the spiritual truths discovered by the ancient Hindus!

At last one man could bear it no more. He had the brain, the power, and the heart—a heart as infinite as the broad sky. He saw how the masses were being led by the priests and how the priests were glorying in their power, and he wanted to do something about it. He did not want any power over anyone, and he wanted to break the mental and spiritual bonds of men. His heart was large. The heart, many around us may have, and we also want to help others. But we do not have the brain; we do not know the ways and means by which help can be given. But this man had the brain to discover the means of breaking the bondage of souls. He learnt why men suffer and he found the way out of suffering. He was a man of accomplishment; he worked everything out. He taught one and all without distinction, and made them realize the peace of enlightenment. This was the man Buddha.

You know from Arnold's poem *The Light of Asia* how Buddha was born a prince and how the misery of the world struck him deeply; how, although brought up and living in the lap of luxury, he could not find comfort in his personal happiness and security; how he renounced the world, leaving his princess and new-born son behind; how he wandered searching for truth from teacher to teacher; and how he at last attained to enlightenment. You know about his long mission, his disciples, his organizations. You all know these things.

Buddha was the triumph in the struggle that had been going on between the priests and the prophets in India. One thing can be said for these Indian priests: they were not and never are intolerant of religion; they never have persecuted religion. Any man was allowed to preach against them—such was their catholicity. They never molested anyone for his religious views. But they suffered from the peculiar weaknesses of all priests: they sought power; they also promulgated rules and regulations and made religion unnecessarily complicated, and thereby undermined the strength of those who followed their religion.

Buddha cut through all these excrescences. He preached the most tremendous truths. He taught the very gist of the philosophy of the Vedas to one and all without distinction; he taught it to the world at large, because one of his great messages was the equality of man. Men are all equal. No concession there to anybody. Buddha was the great preacher of equality. Every man and woman has the same right to attain spirituality—that was his teaching. The difference between the priests and the other castes he abolished. Even the lowest were entitled to the highest attainments; he opened the door of Nirvāna to one and all. His teaching was bold even for India. No amount of preaching can ever shock the Indian soul; but it was hard for India to swallow Buddha's doctrine. How much harder it must be for you!

His doctrine was this: Why is there misery in our life? Because we are selfish. We desire things for ourselves—that is why there is misery. What is the way out? The giving up of the self. The self does not exist; the phenomenal world, all this that we perceive, is all that exists. There is nothing called soul underlying the cycle of life and death. There is a stream of thought, one thought following another in succession, each thought coming into existence and becoming nonexistent at the same moment. That is all. There is no thinker of the thought, no soul. The body is changing all the time; so is mind, consciousness. The self therefore is a delusion. All selfishness comes of holding on to the self, to this illusory self. If we know the truth that there is no self, then we shall be happy and make others happy.

This was what Buddha taught. And he did not merely talk; he was ready to give up his own life for the world. He said, "If sacrificing an animal is good, sacrificing a man is better," and he offered himself as a sacrifice. He said: "This animal sacrifice is another superstition. God and soul are the two big superstitions. God is only a superstition invented by the priests. If there is a God, as these brāhmins preach, why is there so much misery in the world? He is just like me, a slave to the law of causation. If He is not bound by the law of causation, then why does He create? Such a God is not at all satisfactory. If there is a Ruler in heaven who rules the universe according to His sweet will and leaves us all here to die in misery—He never has the kindness to look at us for a moment. Our whole life is continuous suffering. But this is not sufficient punishment: after death we must go to places where we have other punishments. Yet we continually perform all kinds of rites and ceremonies to please this Creator of the world!"

Buddha said: "These ceremonials are all wrong. There is but one ideal in the world. Destroy all delusions; what is true will remain. As soon as the clouds are gone, the sun will shine." How is one to kill the self? Be perfectly unselfish; be ready to give up your life even for an ant. Give up all superstition; work not to please God, to get any reward, but work because you are seeking your own release by killing your self. Worship and prayer and all that—these are all nonsense. You all say, "I thank God"—but where does

He live? You do not know and yet you are all going crazy because of your belief in God.

The Hindus can give up everything except their God. To deny God is to cut the very ground from under the feet of devotion. Devotion and God the Hindus must cling to. They can never relinquish these. And here, in the teaching of Buddha, are no God and no soul—simply work. What for? Not for the self, for the self is a delusion. We shall be free when this delusion has vanished. Very few are there in the world that can rise to that height and work for work's sake.

Yet the religion of Buddha spread fast. It was because of the marvellous love which, for the first time in the history of humanity, overflowed a large heart and devoted itself to the service not only of all men but of all living things—a love which did not care for anything except to find a way of release from suffering for all beings.

Man was loving God and had forgot all about his brother man. The man who in the name of God could give up his life could also turn around and kill his brother man in the name of the same God. That was the state of the world. Men would sacrifice their sons for the glory of God, would rob nations for the glory of God, would kill thousands of beings for the glory of God, would drench the earth with blood for the glory of God. Buddha was the first to turn their minds to the other God—man. It was man that was to be loved. Buddha set in motion the first wave of intense love for all men, the first wave of true, unadulterated wisdom, which, starting from India, gradually inundated country after country—north, south, east, west.

This teacher wanted to make truth shine as truth. No softening, no compromise, no pandering to the priests and the powerful kings. No bowing before superstitious traditions, however hoary; no respect for forms and books just because they came down from the distant past. He rejected all scriptures, all forms of religious practice. Even the very language, Sanskrit, in which religion had been traditionally taught in India, he rejected, so that his followers would not have any chance to imbibe the superstitions which were associated with it.

There is another way of looking at the truth we have been discussing: the Hindu way. We claim that Buddha's great doctrine of selflessness can be better understood if it is looked at in our way. In the Upanishads there was already the great doctrine of Ātman and Brahman. Ātman, the Self, is the same as Brahman, the Lord. This Self is all that is; It is the only Reality. Māyā, delusion, makes us see It as differentiated. There is one Self, not many. That one Self shines in various forms. Man is man's brother because all men are one. A man is not only my brother, say the Vedas, but he is myself. Hurting any part of the universe, I only hurt myself. I am the universe. It is a delusion to think that I am Mr. So-and-so.

The more you approach your Self, the more quickly delusion vanishes. The more all differences and divisions disappear, the more you realize all as the one Divinity. God exists, but He is not a man sitting upon a cloud. He is pure Spirit. Where does He reside? Nearer to you than your very self. He is the Soul. How can you perceive God as separate and different from yourself? When you think of Him as someone separate from yourself, you do not know Him. He is you yourself. That was the doctrine of the prophets of India.

It is selfishness to think that you are Mr. So-and-so and all the world is different from you. You believe that you are different from me. You do not take any thought of me. You go home and have your dinner and sleep. If I die you still eat, drink, and are merry. But you cannot really be happy when the rest of the world is suffering. We are all one. It is the delusion of separateness that is the root of misery. Nothing exists but the Self. There is nothing else.

Buddha's idea was that there was no God, but only man. He repudiated the mentality which underlay the prevalent ideas of God. He found they made men weak and superstitious. If God gives you everything you pray for, why then do you go out and work? God comes to those who work. God helps them that help themselves. An opposite idea of God weakens our nerves, softens our muscles, makes us dependent. Only the independent are happy; and the dependent are miserable. Man has infinite power within himself and he can realize it—he can realize himself as the one, infinite Self. It can be done; but you do not believe it. You pray to God and keep your powder dry all the time.

Buddha taught the opposite. Do not let men weep. Let them have none of this praying and all that. God is not keeping shop. With every breath you are pray- ing to God. I am talking—that is a prayer. You are listening—that is a prayer. Is there ever any move-

ment of yours, mental or physical, in which you do
not make use of the infinite Divine Energy? It is all
a constant prayer. If you call only a set of words prayer,
you make prayer superficial. Such prayers are not
much good; they can scarcely bear any real fruit. Is
prayer a magic formula by repeating which, even if
you do not work hard, you gain miraculous results?
No. All have to work hard; all have to reach the depths
of that Infinite Energy. Behind the poor, behind the
rich, there is the same Infinite Energy. It is not true
that while one man works hard, another by repeating
a few words achieves the same results. This universe
is a constant prayer. If you take prayer in this sense,
I am with you. Words are not necessary. Better is
silent prayer.

The vast majority of people do not understand the
meaning of this doctrine. In India any compromise
regarding the Self means that we have given power
into the hands of the priests and have forgotten the
great teachings of the prophets. Buddha knew this;
so he brushed aside all the priestly doctrines and practices and made man stand on his own feet. It was
necessary for him to go against the accustomed ways
of the people; he had to bring about revolutionary
changes. As a result this sacrificial religion passed away
from India for ever and was never revived.

Buddhism apparently has passed away from India,
but really it has not. There was an element of danger
in the teaching of Buddha: it was a reforming religion.
In order to bring about the tremendous spiritual change
he did, he had to give many negative teachings. But
if a religion emphasizes the negative side too much,

it is in danger of eventual destruction. Never can a reforming sect survive if it is only reforming; the positive elements alone—the real impulse, that is, the principles—live on and on. After a reform has been brought about it is the positive side that should be emphasized; after the building is finished the scaffolding must be taken away.

It so happened in India that as time went on the followers of Buddha emphasized the negative aspect of his teachings too much and thereby caused the eventual downfall of their religion. The positive aspects of truth were suffocated by the forces of negation, and thus India repudiated the destructive tendencies that flourished in the name of Buddhism. That was the decree of the Indian national thought.

The negative ideas of Buddhism—that there is no God and no soul—died out. I can say that God is the only Being that exists; it is a very positive statement. He is the one Reality. When Buddha says there is no soul, I say, "Man, thou art one with the universe; thou art all things." How positive! The reformative element died out, but the formative element has lived through all time. Buddha taught kindness towards lower beings, and since then there has not been a sect in India that has not taught charity to all beings, even to animals. This kindness, this mercy, this charity— greater than any doctrine—are what Buddhism left to us.

The life of Buddha has an especial appeal. All my life I have been very fond of Buddha, but not of his doctrine. I have more veneration for that character than for any other—that boldness, that fearlessness, and that tremendous love. He was born for the good of men. Others may seek God, others may seek truth for themselves; he did not even care to know truth for himself. He sought truth because people were in misery. How to help them—that was his only concern. Throughout his life he never had a thought for himself. How can we ignorant, selfish, narrow-minded human beings ever understand the greatness of this man?

And consider his marvellous brain. No emotionalism. That giant brain never was superstitious. "Believe not because an old manuscript has been produced, because it has been handed down to you from your forefathers, because your friends want you to—but think for yourself; search out truth for yourself; realize it yourself. Then if you find it beneficial to one and all, give it to people." Soft-brained men, weak-minded, chicken-hearted, cannot find the truth. One has to be free and as broad as the sky. One has to have a mind that is crystal clear; only then can truth shine in it. We are so full of superstitions! Even in your country, where you think you are highly educated, how full of narrownesses and superstitions you are! Just think, with all your claims to civilization in this country, on one occasion I was refused a chair to sit on, because I was a Hindu!

Six hundred years before the birth of Christ, at the time when Buddha lived, the people of India must have had wonderful education. Extremely free-minded they must have been. Great masses followed him. Kings gave up their thrones; queens gave up their thrones. People were able to appreciate and embrace his teaching—so revolutionary, so different from what they had been taught by the priests through the ages. Their minds must have been unusually free and broad.

And consider his death. If he was great in life, he was also great in death. He ate food offered to him by a member of a race similar to your American Indians. Hindus do not touch these people because they eat indiscriminately. He told his disciples: "Do not eat this food, but I cannot refuse it. Go to the man and tell him he has done me one of the greatest services of my life: he has released me from the body." An old man came and sat near him—he had walked miles and miles to see the Master—and Buddha taught him. When he found a disciple weeping, he reproved him, saying: "What is this? Is this the result of all my teaching? Let there be no false bondage, no dependence on me, no false glorification of this passing personality. The Buddha is not a person; he is a state of realization. Work out your own salvation."

Even when dying he would not claim any distinction for himself. I worship him for that. What you call Buddhas and Christs are only the names of certain states of realization. Of all the teachers of the world, he was the one who taught us most to be self-reliant, who freed us not only from the bondage of our false selves but from dependence on the invisible Being or beings called God or gods. He invited everyone to enter into that state of freedom which he called Nirvāna. All must attain to it one day, and that attainment is the complete fulfilment of man.

THE GREAT TEACHERS OF THE WORLD

(Delivered at the Shakespeare Club, Pasadena, California, February 3, 1900)

THE UNIVERSE, according to a philosophical theory of the Hindus, is moving in cycles of wave form. It rises, reaches its zenith, and then falls and remains in the hollow, as it were, for some time, once more to rise, and so on in wave after wave. What is true of the universe is true of every part of it. The march of human affairs is like that; the history of nations is like that: they rise and they fall. After the rise comes a fall; again, out of the fall comes a rise, with greater power. This movement is always going on.

In the religious world the same movement exists. In every nation's spiritual life there is a fall as well as a rise. The nation goes down and everything seems to go to pieces. Then again it gains strength and rises. A huge wave comes—sometimes a tidal wave; and always on the crest of that tidal wave is a shining soul, a Messenger. Creator and created by turns, he is the impetus that makes the wave rise, the nation rise; at the same time, he is created by the same forces which make the wave, acting and interacting by turns. He puts forth his tremendous power upon society, and society makes him what he is. These are the great world thinkers; these are the Prophets, the Messengers, the Incarnations of God.

Men have an idea that there can be only one religion,

that there can be only one Prophet, that there can be
only one Incarnation; but that idea is not true. By
studying the lives of all these great Messengers, we
find that each was destined to play a part, as it were,
and a part only; that the true harmony consists in the
sum total and not in one note. It is the same in the
life of races: no race is born to alone enjoy the world.
None dare say so. Each race has a part to play in this
divine harmony of nations; each race has its mission
to perform, its duty to fulfil. The sum total is the
great harmony.

So not one of these Prophets is born to rule the
world for ever. None has yet succeeded and none is
going to succeed in the future. Each only contributes
a part; and he will control the world and its destinies
as far as that part is concerned.

Most of us are born believers in a Personal God.
We talk of principles, we think of theories, and that
is all right; but every thought and every movement,
every one of our actions, shows that we can only
understand a principle when it comes to us through a
person. We can only grasp an idea when it comes to
us through a concrete ideal person. We can only understand the precept through the example. Would to God
that all of us were so developed that we did not require
any example, did not require any persons. But that we
are not; and naturally the vast majority of mankind
have put their souls at the feet of these extraordinary
personalities, the Prophets, the Incarnations of God—
Incarnations worshipped by the Christians, by the
Buddhists, and by the Hindus. The Mohammedans
from the beginning stood out against any such worship.

They would have nothing to do with worshipping the Prophets or the Messengers, or paying any homage to them; but practically, instead of one Prophet, thousands upon thousands of saints are being worshipped. We cannot go against facts. We are bound to worship personalities, and it is good. Remember the answer of your great Prophet to the prayer, "Lord, show us the Father"—"He that hath seen me hath seen the Father." Which of us can have a better idea of God than that He is a man? We can see Him only in and through humanity. The vibration of light is everywhere in this room; why cannot we see it everywhere? You can see it only in the lamp. God is an omnipresent Principle— everywhere; but we are so constituted at present that we can see Him, feel Him, only in and through a human God.

When these great Lights come, then man realizes God. And they come in a different way from the way we come. We come as beggars; they come as emperors. We come here like orphans, as people who have lost their way and do not know it. What are we to do? We do not know what is the meaning of our lives. We cannot realize it. Today we are doing one thing, tomorrow another. We are like little bits of straw drifting to and fro in water, like feathers blown about in a hurricane. But in the history of mankind you will find that these Messengers come, and that from their very birth their mission is found and formed. The whole plan is there, laid down, and you see them swerving not one inch from it.

Because they come with a mission, they come with a message. They do not want to reason. Did you ever hear or read of these great Teachers or Prophets reasoning out what they taught? No; not one of them has done so. They speak direct. Why should they reason? They see the Truth. And not only do they see It, but they show It. If you ask me, "Is there any God?" and I say "Yes," you immediately ask my grounds for saying so, and poor me has to exercise all his powers to provide you with some reason. If you had come to Christ and said, "Is there any God?" he would have said, "Yes"; and if you had asked, "Is there any proof?" he would have replied, "Behold the Lord!" And thus, you see, it is a direct perception, and not at all the ratiocination of logic. There is no groping in the dark; but there is the strength of direct vision. I see this table; no amount of reason can take that faith from me. It is a direct perception. Such is their faith—faith in their ideals, faith in their mission, above all else faith in themselves. The great Shining Ones believe in themselves as nobody else ever does.

The people say: "Do you believe in God? Do you believe in a future life? Do you believe in this doctrine or that dogma?" But here the base is wanting: this belief in oneself. Ay! the man who cannot believe in himself, how can they expect him to believe in anything else? I am not sure of my own existence. One moment I think that I am existing and nothing can destroy me; the next moment I am quaking in fear of death. One minute I think I am immortal; the next minute a spook appears, and then I don't know what I am or where I am; I don't know whether I am living or dead. One moment I think that I am spiritual, that I am moral; and the next moment a blow comes, and

I am thrown flat on my back. And why? I have lost faith in myself; my moral backbone is broken.

But in these great Teachers you will always find this sign: that they have intense faith in themselves. Such intense faith is unique and we cannot understand it. That is why we try to explain away in various ways what these Teachers speak of themselves; and people invent twenty thousand theories to explain what they say about their realization. We do not think of ourselves in the same way, and naturally we cannot understand them.

Then again, when they speak the world is bound to listen. When they speak each word is direct; it bursts like a bombshell. What is in the word unless it has the power behind? What matters it what language you speak and how you arrange your language? What matters it whether or not you speak with correct grammar and fine rhetoric? What matters it whether your language is ornamental or not? The question is whether or not you have anything to give. It is a question of giving and taking, and not of listening. Have you anything to give?—that is the first question. If you have, then give. Words but convey the gift; they are but one of the many modes.

Sometimes they do not speak at all. There is an old Sanskrit verse which says: "I saw the teacher sitting under a tree. He was a young man of sixteen and the disciple was an old man of eighty. The preaching of the teacher was in silence, and the doubts of the doubter departed." Thus, though they do not speak at all, yet they can convey the truth from mind to mind. They come to give. They command—they, the

Messengers; you have to obey the command. Do you not remember in your own scriptures the authority with which Jesus speaks? "Go ye, therefore, and teach all nations, . . . teaching them to observe all things whatsoever I have commanded you." It runs through all his utterances, that tremendous faith in his own message. That you find in the life of all these great giants whom the world worships as its Prophets.

These great teachers are the living Gods on this earth. Whom else should we worship? I try to get an idea of God in my mind, and I find what a false little thing I conceive; it would be a sin to worship that as God. I open my eyes and look at the actual life of these great ones of the earth. They are higher than any conception of God that I could ever form. For what idea of mercy could be formed by a man like me, who would go after a man if he steals anything from me and send him to jail? And what can be my highest idea of forgiveness? Nothing beyond myself. Which of you can jump out of his own body? Which of you can jump out of his own mind? Not one of you. What idea of divine love can you form except what you actually feel? What we have never experienced we can form no idea of. So all my best attempts at forming an idea of God will fail in every case. And here are plain facts and not ideas—actual facts of love, of mercy, of purity, of which I cannot even have any conception. What wonder that I should fall at the feet of these men and worship them as God? And what else can anyone do? I should like to see the man who can do anything else, however much he may talk. Talking is not actuality. Talking about God and the

Impersonal, and this and that, is all very good; but these man-Gods are the real Gods of all nations and all races. These divine men have been worshipped and will be worshipped so long as man is man. Therein is our faith, therein is our hope. Of what avail is a mere mystical principle?

The purpose and intent of what I have to say to you is this: that I have found it possible in my life to worship all of them and to be ready for all that are yet to come. A mother recognizes her son in any dress in which he may appear before her; and if she does not do so, I am sure that she is not the mother of that man. Now, as regards those of you who think you understand Truth and Divinity and God in only one Prophet in the world, and not in any other, naturally, the conclusion which I draw is that you do not understand Divinity in anybody; you have simply swallowed words and identified yourself with one sect, just as you would in party politics, as a matter of opinion. But that is no religion at all. There are some fools in this world who use brackish water although there is excellent sweet water near by, because, they say, the brackish-water well was dug by their father. Now, in my little experience I have collected this knowledge: that for all the devilry that religion is blamed for, religion is not at all at fault. No religion ever persecuted men, no religion ever burnt witches, no religion ever did any of these things. What then incited people to do these things? Politics, but never religion; and if such politics takes the name of religion, whose fault is that?

So when a man stands up and says, "My Prophet is

the only true Prophet," he is not right; he knows not the A B C of religion. Religion is neither talk nor theory nor intellectual consent. It is realization in our heart of hearts; it is touching God; it is feeling, realizing that I am a spirit related to the Universal Spirit and all Its great manifestations. If you have really entered the house of the Father, how can you have seen His children and not know them? And if you do not recognize them, you have not entered the house of the Father. The mother recognizes her child in any dress and knows him however disguised. Recognize all the great spiritual men and women in every age and country and see that they are not really at variance with one another.

Wherever there has been actual religion—this touch of the Divine, the soul coming in direct contact with the Divine—there has always been a broadening of the mind which has enabled it to see the light everywhere. Now, the Mohammedans are the crudest in this respect, and the most sectarian. Their watchword is: "There is one God and Mohammed is His Prophet." Everything beyond that not only is bad but must be destroyed forthwith; at a moment's notice every man or woman who does not exactly believe in that must be killed; everything that does not belong to this worship must be immediately broken; every book that teaches anything else must be burnt. From the Pacific to the Atlantic, for five hundred years, blood ran all over the world. That is Mohammedanism. Nevertheless, among these Mohammedans, wherever there was a philosophic man he was sure to protest against these cruelties. In that he showed the touch of the Divine and realized a fragment of the truth; he was not playing with his religion—for it was not his father's religion he was talking about—but spoke the truth direct, like a man.

Side by side with the modern theory of evolution there is another thing: atavism. There is a tendency in us to revert to old ideas in religion. Let us think something new, even if it be wrong. It is better to do that. Why should we not try to hit the mark? We become wiser through failures. Time is infinite. Look at the wall. Did the wall ever tell a lie? It is always the wall. Man tells a lie—and becomes a god, too. It is better to do something; never mind even if it proves to be wrong. It is better than doing nothing. The cow never tells a lie, but she remains a cow all the time. Do something. Think some thought; it doesn't matter whether you are right or wrong. But think something. Because my forefathers did not think this way, shall I sit down quietly and gradually lose my sense of feeling and my own thinking faculty? I may as well be dead. And what is life worth if we have no living ideas, no convictions of our own, about religion? There is some hope for the atheists, because though they differ from others, they think for themselves. The people who never think anything for themselves are not yet born into the world of religion; they have a mere jelly-fish existence. They will not think; they do not care for religion. But the disbeliever, the atheist, cares and he is struggling. So think something. Struggle Godwards. Never mind if you fail, never mind if you get hold of a queer theory. If you are afraid to be called queer, keep it in your own mind; you need not go out and preach it to others. But do something. Struggle Godwards. Light must come. If a man feeds me every day of my life, in the long run I shall lose the use of my hands. Spiritual death is the result of following others as in a flock of sheep. Death is the result of inaction. Be active; and wherever there is activity there must be difference. Difference is the sauce of life; it is the beauty, it is the art, of everything: difference makes all beautiful here. It is variety that is the source of life, the sign of life. Why should we be afraid of it?

Now we are coming into a position to understand about the Prophets. We see that the historical evidence is—apart from the jelly-fish acceptance of dogmas—that where there has been any real thinking, any real love of God, the soul has grown Godwards and has got, as it were, a glimpse now and then, has attained direct perception, even for a second, even once in its life. Immediately "all doubts vanish for ever, all the crookedness of the heart is made straight, all bondage vanishes, and the results of past actions fly away; for He is seen who is the nearest of the near and the farthest of the far." That is religion; that is all of religion. The rest is mere theory, dogma, so many ways of going to that state of direct perception. Now we are fighting over the basket and the fruits have fallen into the ditch.

If two men quarrel about religion, just ask them the question: "Have you seen God? Have you seen spiritual things?" One man says that Christ is the only Prophet. Well, has he seen Christ? "Has your father seen him?" "No, sir." "Has your grandfather seen him?" "No, sir." "Have you seen him?" "No, sir." "Then what are you quarrelling for? The fruits have fallen into the ditch and you are quarrelling over the basket!" Sensible men and women should be ashamed to go on quarrelling in that way.

These Messengers and Prophets were great and true. Why so? Because each one came to preach a great idea. Take the Prophets of India, for instance. They are the oldest of the founders of religion. We take, first, Krishna. You who have read the Gītā know that the one idea all through the book is non-attachment. Remain unattached. The heart's love is due to only One. To whom? To Him who never changes. Who is that One? He is God. Do not make the mistake of giving the heart to anything that is changing, because that is misery. You may give it to a man; but if he dies, misery is the result. You may give it to a friend; but tomorrow he may become your enemy. If you give it to your husband, he may one day quarrel with you. You may give it to your wife, and she may die the day after tomorrow. Now, this is the way the world is going on. So says Krishna in the Gītā. The Lord is the only one who never changes. His love never fails. Wherever we are and whatever we do, He is ever and ever the same merciful, the same loving Spirit. He never changes, He is never angry, whatever we do.

How can God be angry with us? Your baby does many mischievous things: are you angry with that baby? Does not God know what we are going to be? He knows we are all going to be perfect sooner or later. He has patience, infinite patience. We must love Him and, only in and through Him, everyone that lives. This is the keynote. You must love your wife, but not for your wife's sake. "Never, O Beloved, is the husband loved on account of the husband, but because the Lord is in the husband." The Vedānta philosophy says that even in the love of husband and wife, although the wife is thinking that she is loving the husband, the real attraction is the Lord, who is present there. He is the only attraction; there is no other. But the wife in most cases does not know that it is so; yet ignorantly she is doing the right thing, which is loving the Lord. Only, when one does it ignorantly it may bring pain. If one does it knowingly, that is salvation. This is what our scriptures say. Wherever there is love, wherever there is a spark of joy, know that to be a spark of His presence, because He is Joy, Blessedness, and Love itself. Without Him there cannot be any love.

This is the trend of Krishna's instruction all through. He has implanted that in his race; therefore when a Hindu does anything, even when he drinks water, he says, "If there is virtue in it, let it go to the Lord." The Buddhist says, if he does any good deed, "Let the merit of the good deed belong to the world; if there is any virtue in what I do, let it go to the world, and let the evils of the world come to me." The Hindu— he is a great believer in God—the Hindu says that God is omnipotent and that He is the Soul of all souls everywhere. So he says, "If I give all my virtues unto Him, that is the greatest sacrifice, and they will go to the whole universe."

Now, this is one message. And what is another message of Krishna? "Whosoever lives in the midst of the world, and works, giving up all the fruit of his action unto the Lord, is never touched by the evils of the world. The lotus, born under the water, rises up and blossoms above the water; even so is the man who is engaged in the activities of the world, giving up all the fruit of his activities unto the Lord."

Krishna strikes still another note as a teacher of intense activity. Work, work, day and night, says the Gitā. You may ask: "Then where is peace? If all through life I am to work like a cart-horse and die in harness, what am I here for?" Krishna says: "Yes, you will find peace. Flying from work is never the way to find peace." Throw off your duties if you can and go to the top of a mountain; even there the mind keeps on going—whirling, whirling, whirling. Someone asked a sannyāsin: "Sir, have you found a nice place? How many years have you been travelling in the Himālayas?" "For forty years," replied the sannyāsin. "There are many beautiful spots to select from and to settle down in; why did you not do so?" "Because for these forty years my mind would not allow me to." We all say, "Let us find peace," but the mind will not allow us to do so.

You know the story of the man who caught a Tartar. A soldier was outside the town, and he cried out when he came near the barracks, "I have caught a Tartar." A voice called out, "Bring him in." "He won't come in, sir." "Then you come in." "He won't let me come in, sir!" So, in this mind of ours, we have "caught a Tartar": neither can we quiet it down nor will it let us be quieted down. We have all "caught Tartars." We all say: Be quiet and peaceful and so forth. But every baby can say that and thinks he can do it. How-

ever, that is very difficult. I have tried. I threw overboard all my duties and fled to the tops of mountains;
I lived in caves and deep forests; but all the same, I
had "caught a Tartar," because I had my world with
me all the time. The "Tartar" is what I have in my
own mind; so we must not blame poor people outside.
"These circumstances are good, and these are bad," so
we say, while the "Tartar" is here within. If we can
quiet him down, we shall be all right.

Therefore Krishna teaches us not to shirk our duties,
but to take them up manfully and not think of the
result. The servant has no right to question. The
soldier has no right to reason. Go forward and do not
pay too much attention to the nature of the work you
have to do. Ask your mind if you are unselfish. If you
are, never mind anything; nothing can resist you.
Plunge in. Do the duty at hand. And when you have
done this, by degrees you will realize the truth: "Whosoever in the midst of intense activity finds intense
peace, whosoever in the midst of the greatest peace
finds the greatest activity, he is a yogi, he is a great
soul, he has arrived at perfection."

Now you can see that the result of this teaching is
that all the duties of the world are sanctified. There
is no duty in this world which we have any right to
call menial; and each man's work is quite as good as
that of an emperor on his throne.

Listen to Buddha's message—a tremendous message. It has a place in our heart. Says Buddha: Root
out selfishness and everything that makes you selfish.
Have neither wife, child, nor family. Be not of the
world; become perfectly unselfish. A worldly man

thinks he will be unselfish, but when he looks at the face of his wife it makes him selfish. The mother thinks she will be perfectly unselfish, but she looks at her baby and immediately selfishness comes. So with everything in this world. As soon as selfish desires arise in a man, as soon as he follows some selfish pursuit, immediately the real man is gone; he becomes like a brute, he is a slave, he forgets his fellow men. No more does he say, "You first and me afterwards," but it is "Me first and let every one else look out for himself."

We find that Krishna's message has a place for us. Without that message we cannot move at all. We cannot conscientiously, and with peace, joy, and happiness, take up any duty of our lives without listening to the message of Krishna: "Be not afraid even if there is evil in your work, for there is no work which has no evil." "Leave it unto the Lord, and do not look for the results."

On the other hand, there is a corner in the heart for the other message: Time flies. This world is finite and all misery. With your good food, nice clothes, and your comfortable home, O sleeping man and woman, do you ever think of the millions that are starving and dying? Think of the great fact that it is all misery, misery, misery! Note the first utterance of the child: when it enters into the world, it weeps. That is the fact: the child weeps. This is a place for weeping. If we listen to Buddha, we shall not be selfish.

Behold another Messenger, he of Nazareth. He teaches: "Be ready, for the kingdom of heaven is at hand." I have pondered over the message of Krishna, and am trying to work without attachment; but sometimes I forget. Then, suddenly, comes to me the message of Buddha: "Take care, for everything in the world is evanescent, and there is always misery in this life." I listen to that and I am uncertain which to accept. Then again comes, like a thunderbolt, the message: "Be ready, for the kingdom of heaven is at hand. Do not delay a moment. Leave nothing for tomorrow. Get ready for that final event, which may overtake you immediately, even now." That message, also, has a place, and we acknowledge it. We salute the Christ; we salute the Lord.

And then comes Mohammed, the Messenger of equality. You ask, "What good can there be in his religion?" If there were no good, how could it live? The good alone lives; that alone survives. Because the good alone is strong, therefore it survives. How long does the influence of an impure man endure? Is it not a fact that the pure man's influence lasts much longer? Without doubt, for purity is strength, goodness is strength. How could Mohammedanism have lived had there been nothing good in its teaching? There is much good. Mohammed was the Prophet of equality, of the brotherhood of man, the brotherhood of all Mussulmans.

So we see that each Prophet, each Messenger, has a particular message. When you first listen to that message, and then look at his life, you see his whole life stand explained, radiant.

Now, ignorant fools start twenty thousand theories and put forward, according to their own mental development, explanations to suit their own ideas, and ascribe them to these great teachers. They take their teachings and put their misconstruction upon them. With every great Prophet his life is the only commentary. Look at his life: what he did will bear out the texts. Read the Gitā, and you will find that it is exactly borne out by the life of the Teacher.

Mohammed by his life showed that among Mohammedans there should be perfect equality and brotherhood. There was no question of race, caste, creed, colour, or sex. The Sultan of Turkey may buy a Negro from the mart of Africa and bring him in chains to Turkey; but should he become a Mohammedan and have sufficient merit and abilities, he might even marry the daughter of the Sultan. Compare this with the way in which the Negroes and the American Indians are treated in this country. And what do Hindus do? If one of your missionaries chanced to touch the food of an orthodox person, he would throw it away. Notwithstanding our grand philosophy, you note our weakness in practice; but there you see the greatness of Islām beyond other faiths, showing itself in equality, perfect equality, regardless of race or colour.

Will other and greater Prophets come? Certainly they will come in this world. But do not look forward to that. I should better like that each one of you become a Prophet of this real New Testament, which is made up of all the Old Testaments. Take all the old messages, supplement them with your own realizations, and become a Prophet unto others. Each one of these Teachers has been great; each has left something for us. They have been our Gods. We salute them; we are their servants. And at the same time we salute ourselves; for if they have been Prophets and children of God, we are Prophets also. They reached their perfection and we are going to attain ours now. Remember the words of Jesus: "The kingdom of heaven is at hand." This very moment let every one of us make a staunch resolution: "I will become a Prophet, I will become a Messenger of Light, I will become a child of God, nay, I will become God Himself."

THE RĀMĀYANA

*(Delivered at the Shakespeare Club, Pasadena,
California, January 31, 1900)*

THERE ARE TWO great epics in the Sanskrit language
which are very ancient. Of course, there are hundreds of other epic poems. The Sanskrit language and
literature have come down to the present day, although
for more than two thousand years Sanskrit has ceased
to be a spoken language. I am now going to speak to
you of the two most ancient epics, called the *Rāmāyana* and the *Mahābhārata*. They embody the manners
and customs, the state of society, civilization, and so
forth, of the ancient Indians. The older of these epics
is called the *Rāmāyana,* the Life of Rāma. There was
some poetical literature before this; the greater part
of the Vedas, the sacred books of the Hindus, are
written in a sort of metre; but this book is held by
common consent in India to be the very beginning of
poetry.

The author of the poem was the sage Vālmiki. Later
on a great many poetical stories were ascribed to this
ancient poet, and gradually it became a very general
practice to attribute to his authorship verses that were
not his. Notwithstanding all these interpolations, the
Rāmāyana comes down to us as a very beautiful epic,
without equal in the literature of the world.

There was a young man who could not in any way
support his family. He was strong and vigorous, and

finally became a highway robber; he attacked persons
in the street and robbed them, and with that money
he supported his father, mother, wife, and children.
This went on continually, until one day a great saint
called Nārada was passing by, and the robber attacked
him. The sage asked the robber: "Why are you going
to rob me? It is a great sin to rob human beings and
kill them. What do you incur all this sin for?" The
robber said, "Why, I want to support my family with
this money." "Now," said the sage, "do you think that
they take a share of your sin also?" "Certainly they
do," replied the robber. "Very good," said the sage;
"make me safe by tying me up here, while you go
home and ask your people whether they will share
your sin in the same way as they share the money you
make." The man accordingly went to his father and
asked, "Father, do you know how I support you?" He
answered, "No, I do not." "I am a robber, and I kill
persons and rob them." "What! you do that, my son?
Get away, you outcaste!" He then went to his mother
and asked her, "Mother, do you know how I support
you?" "No," she replied. "Through robbery and mur-
der." "How horrible it is!" cried the mother. "But do
you partake in my sin?" said the son. "Why should I?
I never committed a robbery," answered the mother.
Then he went to his wife and questioned her. "Do
you know how I maintain you all?" "No," she re-
sponded. "Why, I am a highwayman," he rejoined,
"and for years have been robbing people; that is how
I support and maintain you all. And what I now want
to know is whether you are ready to share in my sin."

"By no means. You are my husband, and it is your duty to support me."

The eyes of the robber were opened. "That's the world!" he exclaimed. "Even my nearest relatives, for whom I have been robbing, will not share in my sin." He came back to the place where he had left the sage, unfastened his bonds, fell at his feet, recounted everything, and said: "Save me! What must I do?" The sage said: "Give up your present course of life. You see that none of your family really loves you; so give up all delusions about them. They will share your prosperity, but the moment you have nothing they will desert you. There is none who will share in your evil; but they will all share in your good. Therefore worship Him who alone stands by us whether we are doing good or evil. He alone loves us; true love never betrays, knows no barter, no selfishness."

Then the sage taught him how to worship. And this man left everything and went into a forest. There he went on praying and meditating until he forgot himself so entirely that when ants came and built ant-hills around him, he was quite unconscious of them. After many years had passed, a voice came saying, "Arise, O sage!" Thus aroused he exclaimed, "Sage? I am a robber!" "No more a robber," answered the voice, "but a purified sage art thou. Forget thine old name. Since thy meditation was so deep and great that thou didst not remark even the ant-hills which surrounded thee, henceforth thy name shall be Vālmiki, 'he that was born in the ant-hill.'" So he became a sage.

And this is how he became a poet: One day as this

sage, Vālmiki, was going to bathe in the holy river Ganges, he saw a pair of doves wheeling round and round and kissing each other. The sage looked up and was pleased at the sight, but in a second an arrow whizzed past him and killed the male dove. As the dove fell down on the ground, the female dove went on whirling round and round the dead body of her companion, in grief. At this sight the sage became miserable, and looking round, he saw the hunter. "Thou art a wretch," he cried, "without the smallest mercy. Thy slaying hand would not even stop for love!" "What is this? What am I saying?" the sage asked himself. "I have never spoken in this way before." And then a voice said to him: "Be not distressed: this is poetry that has come out of your mouth. Write the life of Rāma in poetic language for the benefit of the world." That is how the epic was written. The first verse sprang out of pity, from the mouth of Vālmiki, the first poet. And it was after that that he wrote the beautiful *Rāmāyaṅa*.

There was in ancient times an Indian town called Ayodhyā; it exists even in modern times. The province in which it is located is called Oudh, and most of you may have noticed it on the map of India. That was the ancient Ayodhyā. There, in olden times, reigned a king called Daśaratha. He had three queens, but no children by any of them; and like all good Hindus, the king and the queens all went on pilgrimages, fasting and praying, that they might have children; and in good time four sons were born. The eldest of them was Rāma.

Now, as it should be, these four brothers were thor-

oughly educated in all branches of learning. To avoid
future quarrels there was in ancient India a custom
according to which the king in his own lifetime nom-
inated his eldest son as his successor, the *Yuvarāja*, or
"Young King," as he was called.

Now, there was another king, called Janaka, and
this king had a beautiful daughter named Sitā. Sitā
had been found in a field and was really a daughter
of the Earth; she was born without parents. The word
sitā in old Sanskrit means the furrow made by a
plough. In the ancient mythology of India you will
find persons born of one parent only, or persons born
without parents, born of the sacrificial fire, born in the
field, and so on—dropped from the clouds, as it were.
All those sorts of miraculous birth were common in the
mythological lore of India.

Sitā, being the daughter of the Earth, was pure and
immaculate. She was brought up by King Janaka.
When she was of a marriageable age, the king wanted
to find a suitable husband for her.

There was an ancient Indian custom called svayamvara, by which the princesses used to choose husbands.
A number of princes from different parts of the country were invited, and the princess, in splendid array,
with a garland in her hand, and accompanied by a
crier who enumerated the distinctive claims of each of
the royal suitors, would walk in the midst of those
assembled before her and select for her husband the
prince she liked by throwing the garland of flowers
round his neck. They would then be married with
much pomp and grandeur.

There were numbers of princes who aspired to the

hand of Sitā; the test demanded on this occasion was the breaking of a huge bow, called the Haradhanu. The princes put forth all their strength to accomplish this feat, but failed; finally Rāma took the mighty bow in his hands and with easy grace broke it in twain. Thus Sitā selected Rāma, the son of King Daśaratha, for her husband, and they were wedded with great rejoicings. Then Rāma took his bride home, and his old father thought that the time was now come for him to retire and appoint Rāma as Yuvarāja. Everything was accordingly made ready for the ceremony, and the whole country was jubilant over the affair, when the youngest queen, Kaikeyi, was reminded by one of her maid-servants of two promises made to her by the king long ago. At one time she had pleased the king very much, and he had offered to grant her two boons. "Ask any two things in my power and I will grant them to you," he had said, but she had made no request then. She had forgotten all about it; but the evil-minded maid-servant in her employ began to work upon her jealousy with regard to Rāma's being installed on the throne, and insinuated to her how nice it would be for her if her own son should succeed the king, until the queen was almost mad with jealousy. Then the servant suggested to her to ask from the king the two promised boons: by the one, her own son Bharata would be placed on the throne, and by the other, Rāma would be exiled to the forest for fourteen years.

Now, Rāma was the very life of the old king; but when this wicked request was made to his father, the latter felt he could not go back on his word. So he did not know what to do. But Rāma came to the rescue and willingly offered to give up the throne and go into exile so that his father might not be guilty of false-hood. So Rāma went into exile for fourteen years, accompanied by his loving wife Sitā and his devoted brother Lakshmana, who would on no account be parted from him.

The Āryans did not know who the inhabitants of these wild forests were. In those days they called the forest tribes "monkeys"; and some of the so-called "monkeys," if unusually strong and powerful, were called "demons."

So into the forest, inhabited by demons and monkeys, Rāma, Lakshmana, and Sitā went. When Sitā had offered to accompany Rāma, he had exclaimed, "How can you, a princess, face hardships and follow me into a forest full of unknown dangers?" But Sitā had replied: "Wherever Rāma goes, there goes Sitā. How can you talk of 'princess' and 'royal birth' to me? I go with you!" So Sitā went. And the younger brother also went with them. They penetrated far into the forest, until they reached the river Godāvari. On the bank of the river they built little cottages, and Rāma and Lakshmana used to hunt deer and collect fruits. After they had lived thus for some time, one day there came a she-monster. She was the sister of the monster-king of Lankā, the island of Ceylon. Roaming through the forest at will, she came across Rāma, and seeing that he was a very handsome man, fell in love with him at once. But Rāma was the purest of men, and also he was a married man; so of course he could not return her love. In revenge, she went to her brother

Rāvana, the monster-king, and told him all about the beautiful Sitā, the wife of Rāma.

Rāma was the most powerful of mortals; there were no giants or demons, or anybody else, strong enough to conquer him. So the monster-king had to resort to subterfuge. He got hold of another monster, who was a magician, and had him change into a beautiful golden deer; the deer went prancing around about the place where Rāma lived, until Sitā was fascinated by its beauty and asked Rāma to go and capture it for her. Rāma went into the forest to catch the deer, leaving his brother in charge of Sitā. Then Lakshmana laid a circle of fire round the cottage and said to Sitā: "Today I fear that some evil may befall you, and therefore I tell you not to go outside this magic circle. Some danger may befall you if you do." Meanwhile Rāma had pierced the magic deer with his arrow, and immediately the deer changed into the form of the monster and died.

Immediately at the cottage was heard the voice of Rāma, crying, "Oh, Lakshmana, come to my help!" and Sitā said, "Lakshmana, go at once into the forest to help Rāma!" "That is not Rāma's voice," protested Lakshmana. But at the entreaties of Sitā, Lakshmana had to go in search of Rāma. As soon as he had gone away, the monster-king, who had taken the form of a mendicant, stood at the gate and asked for alms. "Wait awhile," said Sitā, "until my husband comes back, and I will give you plentiful alms." "I cannot wait, good lady," said he; "I am very hungry; give me anything you have." At this, Sitā, who had a few fruits in the cottage, brought them out. But the mendicant monk, after much persuading, prevailed upon her to bring the alms to him, assuring her that she need have no fear since he was a holy person. So Sitā came out of the magic circle, and immediately the seeming monk assumed his monster body. Grasping her in his arms, he called his magic chariot and, putting her therein, fled with the weeping Sitā. Poor Sitā! She was utterly helpless; nobody was there to come to her aid. As the monster was carrying her away, she took off a few of the ornaments from her person and at intervals dropped them to the ground.

She was taken by Rāvana to his kingdom, Lankā. He made proposals to her to become his queen, and tempted her in many ways to accede to his request. But Sitā, who was chastity itself, would not even speak to the monster, and he, to punish her, made her live under a tree day and night, until she should consent to be his wife.

When Rāma and Lakshmana returned to the cottage and found that Sitā was not there, their grief knew no bounds. They could not imagine what had become of her. The two brothers went on seeking, seeking everywhere for Sitā, but could find no trace of her. After long searching, they came across a group of monkeys, and in the midst of them was Hanumān, the "divine" monkey. Hanumān, the best of the monkeys, became the most faithful servant of Rāma and helped him in rescuing Sitā, as we shall see later on. His devotion to Rāma was so great that he is still worshipped by the Hindus as the ideal of a true servant of the Lord. You see, by the monkeys and demons were meant the aborigines of Southern India.

So Rāma at last came to these monkeys. They told him that they had seen flying through the sky a chariot in which was seated a demon who was carrying away a most beautiful lady, and that she was weeping bitterly; and as the chariot passed over their heads she dropped one of her ornaments to attract their attention. Then they showed Rāma the ornament. Lakshmana took the ornament and said: "I do not know whose ornament this is." Rāma took it from him and recognized it at once, saying, "Yes, it is Sitā's." Lakshmana could not recognize the ornament because he had never looked upon the arms and the neck of Sitā—such was the reverence in which he held her, his elder brother's wife. So you see, since it was a necklace he did not know whose it was. There is in this episode a touch of the old Indian custom. Then the monkeys told Rāma who this monster-king was and where he lived, and they all went to seek for him.

Now, the monkey-king Vāli and his younger brother Sugriva were then fighting among themselves for the kingdom. The younger brother was helped by Rāma, and he regained the kingdom from Vāli, who had driven him away; and he in return promised to help Rāma. They searched the country all around, but could not find Sitā. At last Hanumān leapt by one bound from the coast of India to Lankā, the island of Ceylon, and went on looking everywhere for Sitā; but nowhere could he find her.

You see, this monster had conquered the gods, men, and in fact the whole world; and he had collected all the beautiful women and made them his concubines. So Hanumān thought to himself: "Sitā cannot be with them in the palace. She would rather die than be in such a place." So Hanumān went to seek for her elsewhere. At last he found Sitā under a tree, pale and thin, like the new moon that lies low on the horizon. Now Hanumān took the form of a little monkey and settled on the tree; and there he witnessed how giantesses sent by Rāvana tried to frighten Sitā into submission, but she would not even listen to the name of the monster-king.

Then Hanumān came nearer to Sitā and told her how he had become the messenger of Rāma, who had sent him to find out where she was; and Hanumān showed Sitā the signet ring which Rāma had given as a token for establishing his identity. He also informed her that as soon as Rāma knew her whereabouts, he would come with an army and conquer the monster and recover her. He suggested to Sitā, however, that if she wished it he would take her on his shoulders and could with one leap clear the ocean and get back to Rāma. But Sitā could not bear the idea, for she was chastity itself and could not touch the body of any man except her husband. So Sitā remained where she was. But she gave him a jewel from her hair to carry to Rāma; and with that Hanumān returned.

Learning everything about Sitā from Hanumān, Rāma collected an army and with it marched towards the southernmost point of India. There Rāma's monkeys built a huge bridge, called Setu-bandha, connecting India with Ceylon.

Now, Rāma was God incarnate; otherwise how could he have done all these things? In India they believe him to be the seventh Incarnation of God.

The monkeys removed whole hills, placed them in the sea, and covered them with stones and trees, thus making a huge embankment. A little squirrel, so it is said, was there, rolling himself in the sand and running backward and forward on to the bridge and shaking himself. Thus in his small way he was working for the bridge of Rāma by putting in sand. The monkeys laughed, for they were bringing whole mountains, whole forests, huge loads of sand for the bridge; they laughed at the little squirrel rolling in the sand and then shaking himself. But Rāma saw it and remarked, "Blessed be the little squirrel; he is doing his work to the best of his ability, and he is therefore quite as great as the greatest of you." Then he gently stroked the squirrel on the back; and the marks of Rāma's fingers running lengthwise are seen on squirrels' backs to this day.

Now, when the bridge was finished the whole army of monkeys, led by Rāma and his brother, entered Ceylon. Tremendous war and bloodshed followed for several months afterwards. At last the monster-king Rāvana was conquered and killed, and his capital, with all the palaces and everything, which were made of solid gold, was taken. In far-away villages in the interior of India, when I tell them that I have been in Ceylon, the simple folk say, "There, as our books tell, the houses are built of gold." So all these golden palaces fell into the hands of Rāma, who gave them over to Vibhishana, the younger brother of Rāvana, and seated him on the throne in place of his brother, in return for the valuable services rendered by him to Rāma during the war.

Then Rāma and Sita were about to leave Lankā.
But there ran a murmur among the followers. "The
test! the test!" they cried. "Sita has not given the test
that she was perfectly pure in Rāvana's household."
"Pure! She is chastity itself!" exclaimed Rāma. "Never
mind! We want the test," persisted the people. Subsequently a huge sacrificial fire was lighted, into which
Sita had to plunge. Rāma was in agony, thinking that
Sita was lost; but in a moment the god of fire himself
appeared, with a throne upon his head, and upon the
throne was Sita. Then there was universal rejoicing
and everybody was satisfied.

Early during the period of exile, Bharata, the
younger brother, had come and informed Rāma of
the death of the old king and earnestly insisted on his
occupying the throne. But Rāma had refused. During
Rāma's exile Bharata would on no account ascend the
throne, and out of respect placed a pair of Rāma's
wooden shoes on it as a substitute for his brother.

Rāma now returned to his capital and by the common consent of his people became the king of
Ayodhyā.

After Rāma regained his kingdom he took the necessary vows which in olden times the king had to take
for the benefit of his people. The king was the servant
of his people and had to bow to public opinion, as
we shall see later on. Rāma passed a few years in
happiness with Sita, when the people again began to
murmur that Sita had been stolen by a demon and
carried across the ocean. They were not satisfied with
the former test and clamoured for another test; otherwise she must be banished.

In order to satisfy the demands of the people, Sitā was banished and left alone in the forest, where was the hermitage of the sage and poet Vālmiki. The sage found poor Sitā weeping and forlorn, and hearing her sad story, sheltered her in his āśrama. Sitā was expecting soon to become a mother, and she gave birth to twin boys. The poet never told the children who they were. He brought them up together in the brahmachārin's life. He then composed the poem known as the *Rāmāyana,* set it to music, and dramatized it.

The drama in India was a very holy thing. Drama and music are themselves held to be religion. Any song—whether it be a love-song or otherwise—if one's whole soul is in that song, leads one to salvation; one has nothing else to do. They say it leads to the same goal as meditation. So Vālmiki dramatized the life of Rāma and taught Rāma's two children how to recite and ·sing it.

There came a time when Rāma was going to perform a huge sacrifice, or yajna, such as kings of old used to perform. But no ceremony in India can be performed by a married man without his wife; he must have his wife with him, the sahadharmini, the "co-partner"—that is the expression for a wife. The Hindu householder has to perform hundreds of ceremonies, but not one can be duly performed, according to the śāstras, if he has not a wife to complement it with her part in it.

Now, Rāma's wife was not with him then, for she had been banished. So the people asked him to marry again. But Rāma for the first time in his life stood against the wishes of the people. He said: "This cannot be. My life is Sitā's." So, as a substitute, a golden statue of Sitā was made, in order that the ceremony could be accomplished. A dramatic entertainment was even arranged to enhance the religious feeling of this great festival. Vālmiki, the great sage-poet, came with his pupils Lava and Kuśa, the unknown sons of Rāma. A stage had been erected and everything was ready for the performance. Rāma and his brothers, attended by all his nobles and his people, made a vast audience. Under the direction of Vālmiki, the life of Rāma was sung by Lava and Kuśa, who fascinated the whole assembly by their charming voices and appearance. Poor Rāma was nearly maddened, and when in the drama the scene of Sitā's exile came about, he did not know what to do. Then the sage said to him, "Do not be grieved, for I will show you Sitā." Then Sitā was brought upon the stage and Rāma was overjoyed to see his wife. All of a sudden the old murmur arose: "The test! the test!" Poor Sitā was terribly overcome by the repeated cruel slight on her reputation; it was more than she could bear. She appealed to mother earth to testify to her innocence, when the earth opened, and Sitā, exclaiming, "Here is the test!" vanished into the bosom of the earth. The people were taken aback at this tragic end, and Rāma was overwhelmed with grief.

A few days after Sitā's disappearance a messenger came to Rāma from the gods, who intimated to him that his mission on earth was finished and he was to return to heaven. These tidings brought to him the recognition of his own real Self. He plunged into the waters of the Sarayu, the mighty river that laved his capital, and joined Sitā in the other world.

This is the great ancient epic of India. Rāma and Sitā are the ideals of the Indian nation. All children, especially girls, worship Sitā. The height of a woman's ambition is to be like Sitā, the pure, the devoted, the all-suffering. When you study these characters you can at once find out how different is the ideal in India from that of the West. For the race, Sitā stands as the ideal of suffering. The West says, "Do: show your power by doing." India says, "Show your power by suffering." The West has solved the problem of how much a man can have; India has solved the problem of how little a man can have—the two extremes, you see. Sitā is typical of India, the idealized India. The question is not whether she ever lived, whether the story is history or not; for we know that the ideal is there. There is no other ideal that has so permeated the whole nation, so entered into its very life, so tingled in every drop of blood of the race, as this ideal of Sitā. Sitā is the name in India for everything that is good, pure, and holy—everything that in woman we call womanly. If a priest has to bless a woman he says, "Be Sitā!" If he blesses a girl he says, "Be Sitā!" They are all children of Sitā and striving to be like Sitā, the patient, the all-suffering, the ever faithful, the ever pure wife. Through all the suffering she experiences, there is not one harsh word against Rāma. She takes it as her own duty and performs her own part in it. Think of the terrible injustice of her being exiled to the forest! But Sitā knows no bitterness. That is, again, the Indian ideal. Says the prophet Buddha:

"When a man hurts you and you turn back to hurt him, that will not cure the first injury; it will only create in the world one more evil." Sitā is a true Indian by nature: she never returns injury.

Who knows which is the truer ideal: the apparent power and strength of the West, or the fortitude in suffering of the East?

The West says, "We minimize evil by conquering it." India says, "We destroy evil by suffering, until evil is nothing to us and becomes positive enjoyment." Well, both are great ideals. Who knows which will survive in the long run? Who knows which attitude will really benefit humanity more? Who knows which will disarm and conquer animality? Will it be suffering or doing?

In the meantime, let us not try to destroy each other's ideals. We are both intent upon the same work, which is the annihilation of evil. You take up your method; let us take up our method. Let us not destroy the ideal. I do not say to the West, "Take up our method." Certainly not. The goal is the same, but the methods can never be the same. And so, after hearing about the ideals of India, I hope that you will say in the same breath to India: "We know the goal is right for us both. You follow your own ideal. You follow your method in your own way, and God speed you!" My mission in life is to ask the East and West not to quarrel over different ideals, but to show them that the goal is the same in both cases, however opposite it may appear. As we wind our way through this mazy vale of life, let us bid each other God-speed.

THE MAHĀBHĀRATA

*(Delivered at the Shakespeare Club, Pasadena,
California, February 1, 1900)*

THE OTHER EPIC, about which I am going to speak to you this evening, is called the *Mahābhārata*. It contains the story of a race descended from King Bharata, who was the son of Dushyanta and Śakuntalā. *Mahā* means great, and *Bhārata* means the descendants of Bharata, from whom India has derived its name, Bhārata. *Mahābhārata* means the Great India or the story of the great descendants of Bharata. The scene of this epic is the ancient kingdom of the Kurus, and the story is based on the great war which took place between the Kurus and the Pāndavas. So the area covered by the epic is not big. This epic is the most popular one in India; and it exercises the same authority in India as Homer's poems did over the Greeks. As ages went on, more and more matter was added to it, until it became a huge book of about a hundred thousand couplets. All sorts of tales, legends, and myths, philosophical treatises, scraps of history, and various discussions were added to it from time to time, until it became a gigantic mass of literature; and through it all runs the old, original story.

The central story of the *Mahābhārata* is about a war between two families of cousins—one family called the Kauravas, the other, the Pāndavas—for empire over India.

The Āryans came into India in small tribes. Gradually these tribes began to spread, until at last they became the undisputed rulers of India; and then arose this fight to gain mastery, between two branches of the same family. Those of you that have studied the Gitā know how the book opens with a description of the battlefield, with two armies arrayed one against the other. That is the war of the *Mahābhārata*.

There were two brothers, sons of an emperor. The elder one was called Dhritarāshtra, and the other was called Pāndu. Dhritarāshtra was born blind. According to Indian law, no blind, halt, maimed, consumptive, or any other constitutionally diseased person can inherit a kingdom. He can only get a maintenance. So Dhritarāshtra could not ascend the throne, though he was the elder son, and Pāndu became the emperor.

Dhritarāshtra had a hundred sons, and Pāndu had only five. After the death of Pāndu at an early age, Dhritarāshtra took charge of the princes and brought up the sons of Pāndu along with his own children. When they grew up they were placed under the tutorship of the great priest-warrior Drona and were well trained in the various martial arts and sciences befitting princes. The education of the princes being finished, Dhritarāshtra put Yudhishthira, the eldest of the sons of Pāndu, on the throne of his father. The sterling virtues of Yudhishthira and the valour and devotion of his other brothers aroused jealousy in the hearts of the sons of the blind king, and at the instigation of Duryodhana, the eldest of them, the five Pāndava brothers were prevailed upon to visit Vāranā-vata on the pretext of a religious festival that was being held there. They were accommodated in a palace made, under Duryodhana's instructions, of hemp, resin, lac, and other inflammable materials, which were subsequently set fire to secretly. But the good Vidura, the step-brother of Dhritarāshtra, having become cognizant of the evil intentions of Duryodhana and his party, had warned the Pāndavas of the plot, and they managed to escape without anyone's knowledge. When the Kurus saw the house reduced to ashes, they heaved a sigh of relief and thought all obstacles were now removed from their path. Then the children of Dhritarāshtra got hold of the kingdom. The five Pāndava brothers had fled to the forest with their mother, Kunti. They lived there by begging and went about in disguise, giving themselves out as brāhmin students. Many were the hardships and adventures they encountered in the wild forests, but their fortitude of mind and their strength and valour enabled them to conquer all dangers. So things went on until they came to hear of the approaching marriage of the princess of a neighbouring country.

I told you last night of a peculiar form of the ancient Indian marriage. It was called svayamvara, that is, the choosing of a husband by a princess. A great gathering of princes and noblemen assembled, from among whom she would choose her husband. Preceded by her trumpeters and heralds, she would approach, carrying a garland of flowers in her hand. At the throne of each candidate for her hand the praises of that prince and all his great deeds in battle would be declared by the heralds. And when the princess decided which prince she desired to have for her husband, she would signify the fact by throwing the marriage garland round his neck. Then the ceremony would turn into a wedding.

King Drupada was a great king, the king of the Pānchālas, and his daughter, Draupadi, famed far and wide for her beauty and accomplishments, was going to choose a husband. At a svayamvara there was always a great feat of arms or something of the kind. On this occasion a mark in the form of a fish was set up high in the sky; under that fish was a wheel with a hole in the centre, continuously turning round, and on the earth below was a tub of water. A man, looking at the reflection of the fish in the water, was to send an arrow and hit the eye of the fish through the chakra, or wheel, and he who succeeded would be married to the princess. Now, there came kings and princes from different parts of India, all anxious to win the hand of the princess, and one after another they tried their skill, and every one of them failed to hit the mark.

You know, there are four castes in India. The highest caste is that of the hereditary priests, the brāhmins; next is the caste of the kshattriyas, composed of kings and fighters; next come the vaiśyas, the traders or business men; and then, the śudras, the servants. This princess was, of course, a kshattriya, one of the second caste.

When all those princes failed in hitting the mark, the son of King Drupada rose up in the midst of the court and said: "The kshattriya, the kingly caste, has failed; now the contest is open to the other castes. Let a brāhmin, even a śudra, take part in it. Whosoever hits the mark marries Draupadi."

Among the brāhmins were seated the five Pāndava brothers. Arjuna, the third brother, was the hero of the bow. He arose and stepped forward. Now, brāhmins as a caste are very quiet and rather gentle people. According to the law, they must not touch a warlike weapon, they must not wield a sword, they must not go into any enterprise that is dangerous. Their life is one of contemplation, study, and control of the inner nature. Judge, therefore, how quiet and peaceable a people they are. When the brāhmins saw this man get up, they thought he was going to bring the wrath of the kshattriyas upon them and they would all be killed. So they tried to dissuade him. But Arjuna did not listen to them, because he was a soldier. He lifted the bow in his hand, strung it without any effort, and drawing it, sent the arrow right through the wheel and hit the eye of the fish.

Then there was great jubilation. Draupadi, the princess, approached Arjuna and threw the beautiful garland of flowers over his head. But there arose a great cry among the princes, who could not bear the idea that this beautiful princess, who was a kshattriya, should be won by a poor brāhmin from among this huge assembly of kings and princes. So they wanted to fight Arjuna and snatch her from him by force. The brothers had a tremendous fight with the warriors, but held their own and carried off the bride in triumph.

The five brothers now returned home to their mother Kunti with the princess. Brāhmins had to live by begging. So since they were living as brāhmins, they used to go out begging, and what they got they brought home and the mother divided it among them. Thus the five brothers, with the princess, came to the cottage where their mother lived. They shouted out to her jocosely, "Mother, we have brought home the most wonderful alms today." The mother replied, "Enjoy it in common, all of you, my children." Then the mother, seeing the princess, exclaimed: "Oh! What have I said? It is a girl!" But what could be done? The mother's word was spoken once for all. It must not be disregarded. The mother's word must be fulfilled. She could not be made to utter an untruth, for she never had done so. So Draupadi became the common wife of all the five brothers.

Now, you know, in every society there are stages of development. Behind this epic there is a wonderful glimpse of the ancient historic times. The author of the poem mentions the fact of the five brothers' marrying the same woman, but he tries to gloss it over, to find an excuse and a cause for such an act: it was the mother's command, the mother sanctioned this strange betrothal, and so on. You know from history that every race has passed through a stage of development which allowed polyandry; all the brothers of a family would marry one wife in common. Now, this is evidently a glimpse of the past, polyandrous stage.

In the meantime the brother of the princess was perplexed in his mind and thought: "Who are these people? Who is this man whom my sister is going to marry? They have not any chariots, horses, or anything. Why, they go on foot!" So he followed them at a distance and at night overheard their conversation and became fully convinced that they were really kshattriyas. Then King Drupada came to know who they were and was greatly delighted.

Though at first many objections were raised, it was declared by Vyāsa that such a marriage was allowable for these princes, and it was permitted. So King Drupada had to yield to this polyandrous marriage, and the princess was married to the five sons of Pāndu.

Then the Pāndavas lived in peace and prosperity and became more powerful every day. Though Duryodhana and his party conceived fresh plots to destroy them, King Dhritarāshtra was prevailed upon by the wise counsels of the elders to make peace with the Pāndavas; and so he invited them home amidst the rejoicings of the people and gave them half of the kingdom. The five brothers built for themselves a beautiful city called Indraprastha, and extended their dominions, laying all the people under tribute to them. Then the eldest, Yudhishthira, in order to declare himself emperor over all the kings of ancient India, decided to perform a Rājasuya Yajna, or Imperial Sacrifice, in which the conquered kings would have to come with tribute and swear allegiance, and help in the performance of the sacrifice by personal service. Śri Krishna, who had become their friend and relative, came to them and approved of the idea. But there was one obstacle to its performance. A king, Jarāsandha by name, who intended to offer a sacrifice of a hundred kings, had eighty-six of them kept as captives with him. Śri Krishna counselled an attack on Jarāsandha; so he, Bhima, and Arjuna challenged the king, who accepted the challenge and was finally conquered by Bhima after fourteen days' continuous wrestling. The captive kings were then set free.

Then the four younger brothers went out with armies on a conquering expedition, each in a different direction, and brought all the kings under subjection to Yudhishthira. Returning, they laid all the vast wealth they had secured at the feet of the eldest brother, to meet the expenses of the great sacrifice.

So to this Rājasuya Sacrifice all the liberated kings came, along with those conquered by the brothers, and rendered homage to Yudhishthira. King Dhritarāshtra and his sons were also invited to come and have a share in the performance of the sacrifice. At the conclusion of the sacrifice, Yudhishthira was crowned emperor and declared lord paramount.

This was the sowing of the future feud. Duryodhana came back from the sacrifice filled with jealousy against Yudhishthira and his brothers; for their sovereignty and vast splendour and wealth were more than he could bear; and so he devised plans to effect their fall by guile, since he knew that to overcome them by force was beyond his power. King Yudhishthira loved gambling, and he was challenged in an evil hour to play dice with Śakuni, the crafty gambler and evil genius of Duryodhana.

In ancient India, if a man of the military caste was challenged to fight, he must at any price accept the challenge to uphold his honour. And if he was challenged to play dice, it was also a point of honour to play, and dishonourable to decline the challenge. King Yudhishthira, says the epic, was the incarnation of all virtues. Even he, the great sage-king, had to accept the challenge.

Śakuni and his party played with loaded dice. So Yudhishthira lost game after game, and stung with his losses, he went on with the fatal play, staking everything he had, and losing all, until all his possessions—his kingdom and everything—were lost. The last stage came when, under a further challenge, he had no other resource left but to stake his brothers, and then himself, and last of all, the fair Draupadi—and lost all. Now they were completely at the mercy of the Kauravas, who cast all sorts of insults upon them and subjected Draupadi to most inhuman treatment. At last, through the intervention of the blind king, they got their liberty and were asked to return home and rule their kingdom.

But Duryodhana saw the danger and forced his father to allow one more throw of the dice, the condition being that the party which would lose must retire to the forests for twelve years and then live unrecognized in a city for one year; but if they were found out, the same term of exile would have to be undergone once again, and then only would the kingdom be restored to the exiles.

This last game Yudhishthira lost also, and the five Pāndava brothers retired to the forests with Draupadi, as homeless exiles. They lived in the forests and mountains for twelve years. There they performed many deeds of virtue and valour, and would go out now and then on a long round of pilgrimages, visiting many holy places. That part of the poem is very interesting and instructive, and various are the incidents, tales, and legends with which it is replete. There are in it beautiful and sublime stories of ancient India, religious and philosophical. Great sages came to see the brothers in their exile and narrated to them many telling stories of ancient India, so as to make them bear lightly the burden of their exile. One only I will relate to you here.

There was a king called Aśvapati. The king had a daughter who was so good and beautiful that she was called Sāvitri, which is the name of a sacred prayer of the Hindus. When Sāvitri grew old enough, her father asked her to choose a husband for herself. These ancient Indian princesses were very independent, as you have already seen, and chose their own princely suitors.

Sāvitri consented and travelled in distant regions, mounted in a golden chariot, with her guards and aged courtiers, to whom her father had entrusted her, stopping at different courts and seeing different princes; but not one of them could win the heart of Sāvitri. They came at last to a holy hermitage in one of those forests that in ancient India were reserved for animals, and where no animals were allowed to be killed. The animals lost their fear of man; even the fish in the lakes came and took food out of the hand. For thousands of years no one had killed anything therein. The sages and the aged went there to live among the deer and the birds. Even criminals were safe there. When a man got tired of life, he would go to the forest, and in the company of sages, talking of religion and meditating thereon, he passed the remainder of his life.

Now, it happened that there was a king, Dyumat-sena, who had been defeated by his enemies and de-prived of his kingdom when he was stricken with old age and had lost his sight. This poor old blind king, with his queen and his son, took refuge in the forest and passed his life in rigid penance. His boy's name was Satyavān.

It came to pass that after having visited all the different royal courts, Sāvitri at last came to this her-mitage, or holy place. Not even the greatest king could pass by the hermitages, or āśramas as they were called, without paying his homage to the sages, such were the honour and respect shown to these holy men. The greatest emperor of India would be only too glad to trace his descent to some sage who lived in a forest, subsisting on roots and fruits, and clad in rags.

So Sāvitri came to this hermitage and saw there Satyavān, the hermit's son, and her heart was con-quered. She had escaped all the princes of the palaces and the courts, but here in the forest refuge of King Dyumatsena, his son Satyavān stole her heart.

When Sāvitri returned to her father's house, he asked her: "Sāvitri, dear daughter, speak. Did you see anybody whom you would like to marry?" Then softly, with blushes, said Sāvitri, "Yes, father." "What is the name of the prince?" "He is no prince, but the son of King Dyumatsena, who has lost his kingdom—a prince without a patrimony, who lives a monastic life, the life of a sannyāsin, in a forest, collecting roots and herbs, helping and feeding his old father and mother, who live in a cottage."

On hearing this the father consulted the sage

Nārada, who then happened to be present there, and he declared it was the most ill-omened choice that was ever made. The king then asked him to explain why it was so. And Nārada said, "Within twelve months from this time the young man will die." Then the king started with terror and spoke: "Sāvitri, this young man is going to die in twelve months and you will become a widow: think of that! Desist from your choice, my child; you shall never be married to a short-lived and fated bridegroom." "Never mind, father; do not ask me to marry another person and sacrifice my chastity of mind, for I love and have accepted in my mind the good and brave Satyavān only as my husband. A maiden chooses only once, and she never departs from her troth." When the king found that Sāvitri was resolute in mind and heart, he complied. Then Sāvitri married Prince Satyavān, and she quietly went from the palace of her father into the forest, to live with her chosen husband and help her husband's parents. Now, though Sāvitri knew the exact date when Satyavān was to die, she kept it hidden from him. Daily he went into the depths of the forest, collected fruits and flowers, gathered faggots, and then came back to the cottage, and she cooked the meals and helped the old people. Thus their lives went on until the fatal day came near, and only three short days remained. She took a severe vow of three nights' penance and holy fasts, and kept her hard vigils. Sāvitri spent sorrowful and sleepless nights with fervent prayers and unseen tears, till the dreaded morning dawned. That day Sāvitri could not bear him out of her sight, even for a moment. She begged permis-

sion from his parents to accompany her husband when
he went to gather the usual herbs and fuel, and gain-
ing their consent, she went. Suddenly, in faltering
accents, he complained to his wife of feeling faint:
"My head is dizzy, and my senses reel, dear Sāvitri.
I feel sleep stealing over me; let me rest beside thee
for a while." In fear and trembling she replied, "Come,
lay your head upon my lap, my dearest lord." And he
laid his burning head in the lap of his wife, and ere
long sighed and expired. Clasping him to her, her
eyes flowing with tears, there she sat in the lonesome
forest, until the emissaries of death approached to take
away the soul of Satyavān. But they could not come
near to the place where Sāvitri sat with the dead body
of her husband, his head resting in her lap. There was
a zone of fire surrounding her, and not one of the
emissaries of death could come within it. They all fled
back from it, returned to King Yama, the god of death,
and told him why they could not obtain the soul of
this man.

Then came Yama, the god of death, the judge of
the dead. He was the first man that had died—the
first man that died on earth—and he had become the
presiding deity over all those that die. He judges
whether, after a man has died, he is to be punished
or rewarded. So he came himself. Of course, he could
go inside that charmed circle, for he was a god. When
he came to Sāvitri he said: "Daughter, give up this
dead body; for know that death is the fate of mortals,
and I am the first of mortals who died. Since then
everyone has had to die. Death is the fate of man."
Thus told, Sāvitri walked off and Yama drew the soul

out. Yama, having possessed himself of the soul of the young man, proceeded on his way. Before he had gone far he heard footfalls upon the dry leaves. He turned back. "Sāvitri, daughter, why are you following me? This is the fate of all mortals." "I am not following thee, Father," replied Sāvitri; "but this is also the fate of woman, that she goes where her love takes her, and the eternal law separates not loving man and faithful wife." Then said the god of death: "Ask for any boon except the life of your husband." "If thou art pleased to grant a boon, O Lord of Death, I ask that my father-in-law may be cured of his blindness and made happy." "Let thy pious wish be granted, duteous daughter." And then the king of death travelled on with the soul of Satyavān. Again the same footfalls were heard from behind. He looked round. "Sāvitri, my daughter, you are still following me?" "Yes, my Father. I cannot help doing so; I am trying all the time to go back, but the mind goes after my husband and the body follows. The soul has already gone, for in that soul is also mine; and when you take the soul, the body follows, does it not?" "Pleased am I with your words, fair Sāvitri. Ask yet another boon of me; but it must not be the life of your husband." "Let my father-in-law regain his lost wealth and kingdom, Father, if thou art pleased to grant another supplication." "Loving daughter," Yama answered, "this boon I now bestow; but return home, for living mortal cannot go with King Yama." And then Yama pursued his way. But Sāvitri, meek and faithful, still followed her departed husband. Yama again turned back. "Noble Sāvitri, follow not in hopeless woe." "I cannot choose but follow where thou takest my loved one." "Then suppose, Sāvitri, that your husband was a sinner and has to go to hell. In that case goes Sāvitri with the one she loves?" "Glad am I to follow where he goes, be it life or death, heaven or hell," said the loving wife. "Blessed are your words, my child. Pleased am I with you. Ask yet another boon; but remember that the dead come not to life again." "Since you so permit me, let the line of my father-in-law not be destroyed; let his kingdom descend to Satyavān's sons." And then the god of death smiled: "My daughter, thou shalt have thy desire now. Here is the soul of thy husband; he shall live again. He shall live to be a father and thy children also shall reign in due course. Return home. Love has conquered death! Woman never loved like thee, and thou are the proof that even I, the god of death, am powerless against the power of the true love that abideth."

This is the story of Sāvitri, and every girl in India must aspire to be like Sāvitri, whose love could not be conquered by death, and who through this tremendous love snatched back even from Yama the soul of her husband.

The book is full of hundreds of beautiful episodes like this. I began by telling you that the *Mahābhārata* is one of the greatest books in the world. It consists of about a hundred thousand verses, in eighteen parvas, or volumes.

To return to our main story. We left the Pāndava brothers in exile. Even there they were not allowed to remain unmolested from the evil plots of Duryodhana; but all of these were futile.

I shall tell you here a story of their forest life. One day the brothers became thirsty in the forest. Yudhishthira bade his brother Nakula go and fetch water. He quickly proceeded in search of a place where there was water and soon came to a lake. He was about to drink of the water, when he heard a voice utter these words: "Stop, my child. First answer my questions, and then drink of this water." But Nakula, who was exceedingly thirsty, disregarded these words, drank of the water, and immediately after dropped down dead. As Nakula did not return, King Yudhishthira told Sahadeva to seek his brother and bring back water with him. So Sahadeva proceeded to the lake and beheld his brother lying dead. Afflicted at the death of his brother, and suffering severely from thirst, he went towards the water, when the same words were heard by him: "My child, first answer my questions, and then drink of the water." He too disregarded these words, and having satisfied his thirst, dropped down dead. Subsequently Arjuna and Bhima were sent, one after the other, on a similar quest, but neither returned, having drunk of the water and dropped down dead. Then Yudhishthira rose up to go in search of his brothers. At length he came to the beautiful lake and saw his brothers lying dead. His heart was full of grief at the sight, and he began to lament. Suddenly he heard the same voice saying: "Do not, my child, act rashly. I am a Yaksha living, as a crane, on tiny fish. It is by me that thy younger brothers have been brought under the sway of the lord of departed spirits. If thou, O Prince, answerest not the questions put by me, even thou shalt become the fifth corpse. Having answered my questions first, do thou, O Kunti's son, drink and carry away as much as thou requirest." Yudhishthira replied: "I shall answer thy questions according to my intelligence. Do thou ask me." The Yaksha then asked him several questions, all of which Yudhishthira answered satisfactorily. One of the questions asked was: "What is the most wonderful fact in this world?" Yudhishthira answered: "We see our fellow beings every moment dying around us, but those who are left think that they will never die. This is the most wonderful fact." Another question was: "How can one know the secret of religion?" And Yudhishthira answered: "By argument nothing can be settled. Doctrines there are many; various are the scriptures, one part contradicting another. There are no two thinkers who do not differ in their opinions. The secret of religion is buried deep, as it were, in dark caves. So the path to be followed is that which the great ones have trodden." Then the Yaksha said: "I am pleased. I am Dharma, the god of justice, in the form of the crane. I came to test thee. Now, thy brothers—see, not one of them is dead. It is all my magic. Since abstention from injury is regarded by thee as higher than both profit and pleasure, therefore let all thy brothers live, O Bull of the Bhārata race." And at these words of the Yaksha, the Pāndavas rose up.

Here is a glimpse of the nature of King Yudhishthira. We can see from his answers that he was more of a philosopher, more of a yogi, than a king.

Now, as the thirteenth year of the exile was drawing nigh, the Yaksha bade them go to Virāt's kingdom and live there in such disguises as they thought best. So after the term of the twelve years' exile had expired, they went to the kingdom of Virāt in different disguises to spend the remaining year in concealment, and entered into menial service in the king's household. Thus Yudhishthira became a brāhmin courtier of the king, as one skilled in dice; Bhima was appointed a cook; Arjuna, dressed as a eunuch, was made a teacher of dancing and music to Uttarā, the princess, and remained in the inner apartments of the king; Nakula became the keeper of the king's horses; Sahadeva got the charge of the cows; and Draupadi, disguised as a lady-in-waiting, was also admitted into the queen's household. Thus concealing their identity, the Pāndava brothers safely spent a year, and the search of Duryodhana to find them out was of no avail. They were only discovered just when the year was out.

Then Yudhishthira sent an ambassador to Dhritarāshtra and demanded that half of the kingdom should, as their share, be restored to them. But Duryodhana hated his cousins and would not consent to their legitimate demands. They were even willing to accept a single province—nay, even five villages. But the headstrong Duryodhana declared that he would not yield without a fight even as much land as a needle's point would hold. Dhritarāshtra pleaded again and again for peace, but all in vain. Krishna also went and tried to avert the impending war and death of kinsmen, as did the wise elders of the royal court; but all negotiations for a peaceful partition of the kingdom were futile. So at last preparations were made on both sides for war, and all the warlike nations took part in it.

In this war the old Indian customs of the kshattriyas were observed. Duryodhana took command of one side; Yudhishthira, of the other. From Yudhishthira messengers were at once sent to all the surrounding kings, entreating their alliance, since honourable men would grant the request that first reached them. So warriors from all parts assembled to espouse the cause of either the Pāndavas or the Kurus, according to the precedence of their requests; and thus one brother joined this side, and the other that side, the father was on one side, and the son on the other. The most curious thing was the code of war of those days: As soon as the battle for the day ceased and evening came, the opposing parties were good friends; they visited each other's tents; but when the morning came, again they proceeded to fight each other. That was the strange trait that the Hindus carried down to the time of the Mohammedan invasion. Then again, a man on horseback must not strike one on foot, must not poison his weapon, must not vanquish the enemy in any unequal fight or by dishonesty, must never take undue advantage of another, and so on. If any deviated from these rules he would be covered with dishonour and shunned. The kshattriyas were trained in that way. And when the foreign invasion came from Central Asia, the Hindus treated the invaders in the self-same way. They defeated them several times, and on as many occasions sent them back to their homes with presents, and so on. The code laid down was that they must not usurp anybody's country; and when a man was beaten, he must be sent back to his country with due regard to his position. The Mohammedan conquerors treated the Hindu kings differently, and when they beat them once, they destroyed them without remorse.

Mind you, in those days—in the times of our story —the poem says, the science of arms was not the mere use of plain bows and arrows; it was magic archery in which the use of mantras, incantations, and so on, played a prominent part. One man could fight millions of men and burn them at will. He could send one arrow, and it would rain thousands of arrows, and thunder; he could make anything burn, and so on. It was all sheer magic. One fact is most curious in both these poems—the *Rāmāyana* and the *Mahābhārata*: along with these magic arrows and all these things going on, you see the cannon already in use. The cannon is an old, old thing, used by the Chinese and the Hindus. Upon the walls of the cities were hundreds of curious weapons made of hollow iron tubes, which, filled with powder and ball, would kill hundreds of men. The people believed that the Chinese, by magic, put the devil inside a hollow iron tube, and when they applied a little fire to a hole, the devil came out with a terrific noise and killed many people.

So in those old days they used to fight with magic arrows. One man would be able to fight millions of others. They had their military arrangements and tactics. There were the foot-soldiers, termed the pada; then the cavalry, the turaga; and two other divisions which the moderns have lost and given up: there was the elephant corps—hundreds and hundreds of elephants, with men on their backs, formed into regiments and protected with huge sheets of iron mail—and these elephants would bear down upon a mass of the enemy. Then there were, of course, the chariots. You have all seen pictures of those old chariots; they were used in every country. These were the four divisions of the army in those old days.

Now, both parties alike wished to secure the alliance of Krishna. But he declined to take an active part and fight in this war, and offered himself as charioteer to Arjuna and as friend and counsellor of the Pāndavas, while to Duryodhana he gave his army of mighty soldiers.

Then was fought on the vast plain of Kurukshetra the great battle in which Bhishma, Drona, Karna, and the brothers of Duryodhana, with the kinsmen on both sides, and thousands of other heroes, fell. The war lasted eighteen days. Indeed, out of the eighteen akshauhinis[1] of soldiers very few men were left. The death of Duryodhana ended the war in favor of the Pāndavas. It was followed by the lament of Gāndhāri, the queen, and the widowed women, and by the funerals of the deceased warriors.

The greatest episode of the war was the marvellous and immortal poem of the Gitā, the Song Celestial. It is the popular scripture of India and the loftiest of all teachings. It consists of a dialogue held by Arjuna with Krishna, just before the commencement of the fight on the battlefield of Kurukshetra. I would advise

[1] An akshauhini is an army division consisting of 21,870 chariots, as many elephants, 65,610 horses, and 109,350 foot-soldiers.

those of you who have not read this book to read it. If you only knew how much it has influenced even your own country! If you want to know the source of Emerson's inspiration, you will find it in the Gitā. He went to see Carlyle, and Carlyle made him a present of the Gitā, and that little book is responsible for the Concord Movement. All the broad movements in America, in one way or other, are indebted to the Concord group.

The central figure of the Gitā is Krishna. As you worship Jesus of Nazareth as God come down as man, so the Hindus worship many Incarnations of God. They believe in not one or two only, but in many, who have come down from time to time, according to the needs of the world, for the preservation of dharma and the destruction of wickedness. Each sect has one, and Krishna is one of them. Krishna perhaps has a larger number of followers in India than any other Incarnation of God. His followers hold that he was the most perfect of these Incarnations. Why? "Because," they say, "look at Buddha and other Incarnations: they were only monks, and they had no sympathy for married people. How could they have? But look at Krishna: He was great as a son, as a king, as a father, and all through his life he practised the marvellous teachings which he preached: 'He who in the midst of the greatest activity finds the sweetest peace, and in the midst of the greatest calmness is most active, he has known the secret of work.' " Krishna shows the way to do this: by being non-attached—doing everything but not being identified with anything. You are the Soul, the Pure, the Free, all the time; you are the Witness. Our misery comes, not from work, but from our getting attached to something. Take, for instance, money. Money is a great thing to have; earn it, says Krishna, struggle hard to get money, but don't get attached to it. So with children, with wife, husband, relatives, fame, everything: you have no need to shun them; only don't get attached. There is only one thing that you should be attached to, and that is the Lord. Work for all, love all, do good to all, sacrifice a hundred lives, if need be, for them, but never be attached. Krishna's own life was the exact exemplification of that.

The book which delineates the life and exploits of Krishna is several thousand years old, and some parts of his life are very similar to that of Jesus of Nazareth. Krishna was of royal birth. There was a tyrant king, called Kamśa, who came to hear of a prophecy that one born of a certain family would occupy his throne. So Kamśa ordered all the male children to be massacred. The father and mother of Krishna were cast by King Kamśa into prison, where the child was born. A light suddenly shone in the prison and the child said, "I am the Light of the world, born for the good of the world." You find Krishna, again, symbolically represented with cows—"The Great Cowherd," as he is called. Sages affirmed that God Himself was born, and they went to pay him homage. In other parts of the story the similarity between the two does not continue.

Śri Krishna conquered the tyrant Kamśa, but he never thought of accepting or occupying the throne himself. He had nothing to do with that. He had done his duty and there it ended.

After the conclusion of the Kurukshetra war, the great warrior and venerable grandsire Bhishma, who fought ten days out of the eighteen days' battle, still lay on his death-bed and gave instructions to Yudhishthira on various subjects, such as the duties of the king, the duties of the four castes, the four stages of life, the laws of marriage, the bestowing of gifts, and so on, basing them on the teachings of the ancient sages. He explained the Sāmkhya philosophy and the Yoga philosophy and narrated numerous tales and traditions about saints and gods and kings. These teachings occupy nearly one fourth of the entire work and form an invaluable storehouse of Hindu laws and moral codes, and so on. Yudhishthira had in the meantime been crowned king. But the awful bloodshed and extinction of superiors and relatives weighed heavily on his mind; and then, under the advice of Vyāsa, he performed the Aśvamedha sacrifice.

After the war, for fifteen years Dhritarāshtra dwelt in peace and honour, obeyed by Yudhishthira and his brothers. Then the aged monarch, leaving Yudhishthira on the throne, retired to the forest with his devoted wife and Kunti, the mother of the Pāndava brothers, to pass his last days in asceticism.

Thirty-six years had now passed since Yudhishthira had regained his empire. Then came to him the news that Krishna had left his mortal body. Krishna, the sage, his friend, his prophet, his counsellor, had departed. Arjuna hastened to Dwārakā and came back only to confirm the sad news that Krishna and the Yādavas were all dead. Then the king and the other brothers, overcome with sorrow, declared that the time for them to go, too, had arrived. So they cast off the burden of royalty, placed Parikshit, the grandson of Arjuna, on the throne, and retired to the Himālayas on the Great Journey, the Mahāprasthāna. This was a peculiar form of sannyāsa. It was a custom for old kings to become sannyāsins. In ancient India, when men became very old, they would give up everything; and so did the kings. When a man did not want to live any more, he then went towards the Himālayas, without eating or drinking, and walked on and on till the body failed. All the time thinking of God, he just marched on till the body gave way.

Then came the gods and the sages, and they told King Yudhishthira that he should go to heaven. To go to heaven one has to cross the highest peaks of the Himālayas. Beyond the Himālayas is Mount Meru. On the top of Mount Meru is heaven. None ever went there in the physical body. There the gods reside. And Yudhishthira was called upon by the gods to go there.

So the five brothers and their wife clad themselves in robes of bark and set out on their journey. On the way they were followed by a dog. On and on they went, and they turned their weary feet northward to where the Himālayas lift their lofty peaks, and they saw the mighty Mount Meru in front of them. Silently they walked on in the snow, until suddenly the queen fell, to rise no more. To Yudhishthira, who was leading the way, Bhima, one of the brothers, said, "Behold, O King, the queen has fallen." The king shed tears, but he did not look back. "We are going to meet Krishna," he said. "No time to look back. March on."

After a while, again Bhima said, "Behold, our brother Sahadeva has fallen." The king shed tears, but paused not. "March on," he cried.

One after the other, in the cold and snow, all four of his brothers dropped down; but unshaken, though alone, the king moved onward. Looking behind, he saw the faithful dog still following him. And so the king and the dog went on, through snow and ice, over hill and dale, climbing higher and higher till they reached Mount Meru; and there they began to hear the chimes of heaven, and celestial flowers were showered upon the virtuous king by the gods. Then descended the chariot of the gods, and Indra said to him, "Ascend in this chariot, greatest of mortals, thou who alone art permitted to enter heaven without changing the mortal body."

But no; that Yudhishthira would not do without his devoted brothers and his queen. Then Indra explained to him that they had already gone thither before him.

Yudhishthira looked around and said to his dog, "Get into the chariot, child." The god stood aghast. "What! The dog?" he cried. "Do thou cast off this dog. The dog goeth not to heaven. Great King, what dost thou mean? Art thou mad? Thou, the most virtuous of men, thou only canst go to heaven in thy physical body." "But he has been my devoted companion through snow and ice. When all my brothers were dead, my queen dead, he alone never left me. How can I leave him now?" "There is no place in heaven for dogs. This dog has to be left behind. There is nothing unrighteous in this." "I do not go to heaven," replied the king, "without the dog. I shall never give up such a one, who has taken refuge with me, until my own life is at an end. I shall never swerve from righteousness, nay, not even for the joys of heaven or the urging of a god." "Then," said Indra, "on one condition the dog goes to heaven. You have been the most virtuous of mortals and he has been a dog, killing and eating animals; he is sinful; he hunted and took other lives. You can exchange heaven with him." "Agreed," said the king. "Let the dog go to heaven."

At once the scene changed. Hearing these noble words of Yudhishthira, the dog revealed himself as Dharma. Dharma is none other than Yama, the lord of death and justice. And Dharma exclaimed: "Behold, O King, no man was ever so unselfish as thou, willing to exchange heaven with a little dog, for his sake disclaiming all his virtues, and ready to go to hell even for him. Thou art well born, O King of kings. Thou hast compassion for all creatures, O Bhārata, of which this is a bright example. Hence regions of undying felicity are thine. Thou hast won them, O King, and thine is a celestial and high reward."

Then Yudhishthira, with Indra, Dharma, and other gods proceeds to heaven in a celestial car. He undergoes some trials, bathes in the celestial Ganges, and assumes a celestial body. He meets his brothers and his wife, who are now immortals, and all at last is bliss.

Thus ends the story of the *Mahābhārata,* setting forth in a sublime poem the triumph of virtue and defeat of vice.

In speaking of the *Mahābhārata* to you, it is simply impossible for me to present the unending array of the grand and majestic characters of the mighty heroes depicted by the genius and master mind of Vyāsa. The internal conflicts between righteousness and filial affection in the mind of the god-fearing yet feeble old blind King Dhritarāshtra; the majestic character of the grand-sire Bhishma; the noble and virtuous nature of the royal Yudhishthira and of the other four brothers, as mighty in valour as in devotion and loyalty; the peerless character of Krishna, unsurpassed in human wisdom; and not less brilliant, the characters of the women: the stately Queen Gāndhāri, the loving mother Kunti, the ever devoted and all-suffering Draupadi—these and hundreds of other characters of this epic, and those of the *Rāmāyana,* have been the cherished heritage of the whole Hindu world for the last several thousands of years and form the basis of its thoughts and of its moral and ethical ideas. In fact, the *Rāmāyana* and the *Mahābhārata* are the two encyclopaedias of the ancient Āryan life and wisdom, portraying an ideal civilization which modern society has yet to aspire after.

GLOSSARY

GLOSSARY

 āchārya   Religious teacher.

Ādityas   Twelve deities (suns) constituting a group.

Advaita   Non-duality; a school of Vedānta philosophy teaching the oneness of God, soul, and universe, whose chief exponent was Śankarāchārya (A.D. 788-820).

ahimsā   Non-injury.

ākāśa   The first of the five material elements that constitute the universe; often translated as "space" and "ether." The four other elements are vāyu (air), agni (fire), ap (water), and prithivi (earth).

animā   Minuteness; one of the supernatural powers, by which a yogi can make himself as small as an atom.

antahkarana   The inner organ; the mind.

Antaryāmin   The Inner Controller.

Arjuna   A hero of the epic *Mahābhārata* and a friend and disciple of Krishna. See Pāndavas.

āśrama   Hermitage; also any one of the four stages of life: the celibate student stage (brahmacharya), the married householder stage (gārhasthya), the stage of retirement and contemplation (vānaprastha), and the stage of religious mendicancy (sannyāsa).

Aśvamedha   The Horse Sacrifice, performed by Hindu kings in ancient India.

Atharva-Veda   One of the four Vedas. See Vedas.

Ātman   The Self or Soul; denotes both the Supreme Soul and the individual soul, which, according to Non-dualistic Vedānta, are ultimately identical.

Avatāra   Incarnation of God.

Ayodhyā   Rāma's capital in North India.

Bhagavad Gitā   An important Hindu scripture, comprising eighteen chapters of the epic *Mahābhārata* and containing the teachings of Śri Krishna.

Bhagavān   The Lord; also used as a title of celebrated saints.

Bhāgavata (*Purāna*)   A well-known scripture dealing mainly with the life and teachings of Krishna.

bhakta   Devotee of God.

bhakti   Love of God.

bhakti-yoga   The path of devotion followed by dualistic worshippers.

bhakti-yogi   A follower of the path of devotion.

Bharata   The son of Śakuntalā and Dushyanta. After him India was named Bhārata or Bhāratavarsha. Also the name of the second brother of Rāma.

Bhārata   A descendent of King Bharata. In the Gitā the word refers occasionally to Dhritarāshtra and frequently to Arjuna, both of whom were descended from the ancient King Bharata.

bhāshya   Commentary.

Bhima   The second son of Pāndu. See Pāndavas.

Bhishma   A hero of the *Mahābhārata* celebrated for his devotion to truth.

Brahmā   The Creator God; the First Person of the Hindu Trinity, the other two being Vishnu and Śiva.

brahmachārin   A celibate student belonging to the first stage of life. See āśrama.

brahmacharya   The first of the four stages of life; the life of an unmarried student. See āśrama.

Brahmaloka   The plane of Brahmā, roughly corresponding to the highest heaven of the dualistic religions, where fortunate souls go after death and enjoy communion with the Personal God.

Brahman   The Absolute; the Supreme Reality of the Vedānta philosophy.

Brahma Sutras An authoritative treatise on the Vedānta philosophy, ascribed to Vyāsa.

brāhmin A member of the priestly caste, the highest caste in Hindu society.

chitta The mind-stuff; that part of the inner organ which is the storehouse of memory or which seeks for pleasurable objects.

Daśaratha The father of Rāma.

devas (Lit., shining ones.) The gods of Hindu mythology.

dharma Righteousness, duty; the inner constitution of a thing, which governs its growth.

Dhritarāshtra An important character in the *Mahābhārata*.

Draupadi The wife of the five Pāndava brothers.

Drona A military teacher mentioned in the *Mahābhārata*.

Drupada The father of Draupadi.

Duryodhana The eldest son of Dhritarāshtra.

Dwārakā A town in Bombay Presidency, associated with Krishna.

Dyāvā-prithivi Sky and earth.

Gāndhāri The mother of Duryodhana.

Gautama A name of Buddha.

Gitā Same as Bhagavad Gitā.

gopis The cowherd girls of Vrindāvan, playmates of Krishna.

gunas A term of the Sāmkhya philosophy, according to which prakriti (nature or matter) consists of three gunas—usually translated as "qualities"—known as sattva, rajas, and tamas. Tamas stands for inertia, rajas for activity or restlessness, and sattva for balance or wisdom.

guru Spiritual preceptor.

Hanumān The great monkey devotee of Rāma, mentioned in the *Rāmāyana*.

Hari An epithet of Vishnu, or the Godhead.

Hiranyagarbha (Lit., the Golden Germ or the Golden Womb.) The first manifestation of Saguna Brahman, or Brahman with attributes, in the relative universe.

Indra The king of the gods.

indriyas The sense-organs, consisting of the five organs of perception, the five organs of action, and the mind.

Iśāna A ruler; an epithet of Śiva and of Vishnu.

Ishta The aspect of the Godhead which a devotee selects as his Chosen Ideal.

Ishta-nishthā Single-minded devotion to the Chosen Ideal.

Iśvara The Personal God.

Janaka A king in Hindu mythology who was endowed with the Knowledge of Brahman.

Jānaki Sitā, the consort of Rāma.

jiva (Lit., living being.) The individual soul, which in essence is one with the Universal Soul.

jivanmukta One who has attained liberation while living in the body.

jivanmukti Liberation while living in the body.

jnāna Knowledge of Reality arrived at through reasoning and discrimination; also the process of reasoning by means of which Ultimate Truth is realized.

jnāna-yoga A form of spiritual discipline mainly based upon philosophical discrimination between the real and the unreal, and renunciation of the unreal.

jnāna-yogi A follower of jnāna-yoga.

jnāni One who follows the path of reasoning and discrimination to realize Ultimate Truth; generally used to denote a non-dualist.

Kaikeyi   A wife of Daśaratha.

karma   Action in general; duty. The Vedas use the word chiefly to denote ritualistic worship and humanitarian action.

karma-yoga   A spiritual discipline, mainly discussed in the Bhagavad Gitā, based upon the unselfish performance of duty.

karma-yogi   A follower of karma-yoga.

karmis   Believers in the Vedic rituals.

Krishna   An Incarnation of God described in the *Mahābhārata* and the *Bhāgavata*.

Kshatra   A member of the warrior race; same as kshattriya.

kshattriya   A member of the second or warrior caste in Hindu society.

Kunti   The mother of the five Pāndava brothers.

Lakshmana   A brother of Rāma.

Lankā   Ceylon.

Madhvāchārya   The chief exponent of Dualistic Vedānta (A.D. 1199-1276).

Mahābhārata   A celebrated Hindu epic.

Mahanirvāna Tantra   One of the principal Tantras. The Tantras are systems of religious philosophy in which the Divine Mother, or Power, and Siva, or the Absolute, are regarded as Ultimate Reality.

mahāpurusha   Great soul.

mahat   The cosmic mind.

manas   The faculty of doubt and volition; sometimes translated as "mind."

mantra   Sacred word by which a spiritual teacher initiates his disciple; Vedic hymn; sacred word in general.

māyā   A term of the Vedānta philosophy denoting ignorance obscuring the vision of Reality; the cosmic illusion
on account of which the One appears as many, the
Absolute as the relative.

Meru   A mythical mountain abounding in gold and
precious stones. The abode of Brahmā, the Creator, and
a meeting-place for the gods, demigods, rishis, and other
supernatural beings, Meru is regarded as the axis around
which the planets revolve.

moksha   Liberation or emancipation, which is the final
goal of life.

mrityu   Death.

mukti   Liberation from the bondage of the world, which
is the goal of spiritual practice.

Nakula   See Pāndavas.

Nārada   A saint in Hindu mythology.

Nārāyana   An epithet of Vishnu, or the Godhead.

"Neti, neti"   (Lit., "Not this, not this.") The negative
process of discrimination, advocated by the followers of
Non-dualistic Vedānta.

Nirvāna   Final absorption in Brahman, or the All-pervading Reality, through the annihilation of the individual ego.

nishthā   Single-minded devotion.

nivritti   Renunciation or detachment.

Nyāya   Indian Logic, one of the six systems of orthodox
Hindu philosophy. It was founded by Gautama.

Om   The most sacred word of the Vedas; also written
Aum. It is a symbol both of the Personal God and of
the Absolute.

pāda   Section.

Pāndavas   The five sons of Pāndu: King Yudhishthira,

Arjuna, Bhima, Nakula, and Sahadeva. They are some of the chief heroes of the *Mahābhārata*.

Pāndu The younger brother of Dhritarāshtra and father of the Pāndavas.

parā Higher.

parā-bhakti Supreme love of the Lord, characterized by complete selflessness.

paramahamsa One belonging to the highest order of sannyāsins.

Parjanya Rain-cloud; the god of rain.

Patanjali The author of the Yoga system, one of the six systems of orthodox Hindu philosophy, dealing with concentration and its methods, control of the mind, and similar matters.

pitris Forefathers.

Prahlāda The young son of the wicked demon king Hiranyakaśipu, who nevertheless developed supreme devotion to God.

prakriti Primordial nature; the material substratum of the creation, consisting of sattva, rajas, and tamas.

prāna The vital breath which sustains life in a physical body; the primal energy or force, of which other physical forces are manifestations.

pratika Substitute.

pratimā Image.

pravritti Desire.

Purānas Books of Hindu mythology.

rajas The principle of restlessness or activity in nature. See gunas.

Rājasuya Yajna A sacrifice mentioned in the Hindu scriptures, performed by an emperor.

rāja-yoga A system of yoga ascribed to Patanjali, dealing with concentration and its methods, control of the mind, samādhi, and similar matters.

rāja-yogi One who follows the disciplines of rāja-yoga.

Rāma The hero of the *Rāmāyana,* regarded by the Hindus as a divine Incarnation.

Ramakrishna A great saint of Bengal, regarded as a Divine Incarnation (A.D. 1836-1886).

Rāmānuja Same as Rāmānujāchārya.

Rāmānujāchārya A great saint of Southern India (A.D. 1017-1137), the foremost interpreter of the school of Qualified Non-dualistic Vedānta, according to which the soul and nature are modes of Brahman, and the individual soul is a part of Brahman.

Rāmāyana A famous Hindu epic.

Rāvana The monster-king of Ceylon, who forcibly abducted Sitā, the wife of Rāma.

Rig-Veda One of the four Vedas. See Vedas.

Rudra An epithet of Śiva.

Sahadeva See Pāndavas.

samādhi Ecstasy, trance, communion with God.

samashti Totality; the universal.

Sāma-Veda One of the four Vedas. See Vedas.

Sāmkhya One of the six systems of orthodox Hindu philosophy, which teaches that the universe evolves as the result of the union of prakriti (nature) and Purusha (Spirit). It was founded by Kapila.

samskāra Mental impression or tendency created by an action.

Śandilya A sage who wrote aphorisms on bhakti, or divine love.

Śankara Same as Śankarāchārya.

Śankarāchārya One of the greatest saints and philosophers of India, the foremost exponent of Advaita Vedānta (A.D. 788-820).

sannyāsa The monastic life; the last of the four stages of life. See āśrama.

sannyāsin A Hindu monk who has renounced the world in order to realize God.

śāntih   Peace.

śāstra   Scripture; sacred book; code of laws.

Satchidānanda   (Lit., Existence-Knowledge-Bliss Absolute.) A name of Brahman, or Ultimate Reality.

sattva   The principle of balance or righteousness in nature. See gunas.

sāttvikas   Those in whom the quality of sattva is greatly developed.

siddha-guru   A teacher who has attained perfection in the spiritual life.

śishya   Disciple.

Sitā   The wife of Rāma.

Śiva   The Destroyer God; the Third Person of the Hindu Trinity, the other two being Brahmā and Vishnu.

Smriti   The sacred books of the Hindus subsidiary to the Vedas, guiding their daily life and conduct; they include the epics, the Purānas, and the *Manu-samhitā* or Code of Manu.

soma   A creeper whose juice was used in Vedic sacrifices.

Sphota   The idea that flashes in the mind when a sound is uttered.

Śri   The word is often used as an honorific prefix to the names of deities and eminent persons, or of celebrated books generally of a sacred character; sometimes used as an auspicious sign at the commencement of letters, manuscripts, etc., or as an equivalent of the English term *Mr*. Also a name of Lakshmi, the Goddess of Fortune.

Śruti   (Lit., hearing.) The Vedas, which in ancient India were transmitted orally from teacher to disciple.

śudra   A member of the fourth or labouring caste in Hindu society.

Śuka   The narrator of the *Bhāgavata* and son of Vyāsa, regarded as one of India's ideal monks.

sutra   Aphorism.

svayamvara   The choosing of a husband by a princess in ancient India.

Swami   (Lit., lord.) A title of the monks belonging to the Vedānta school.

tamas   The principle of dullness or inertia in nature. See gunas.

Tantra   A system of religious philosophy in which the Divine Mother, or Power, and Śiva, or the Absolute, are regarded as Ultimate Reality.

Tulsidās   A celebrated Vaishnava poet and author of the version of the *Rāmāyana* associated with his name.

Upanishads   The well-known Hindu scriptures containing the philosophy of the Vedas. They are one hundred and eight in number, of which eleven are called major Upanishads.

vairāgya   Renunciation.

Vaishnavas   The followers of Vishnu; a dualistic sect which emphasizes the path of devotion as a spiritual discipline.

vaiśya   A member of the third caste in Hindu society, which engages in agriculture, commerce, and cattle-rearing.

Vālmiki   The author of the *Rāmāyana*.

vānaprasthin   One who has entered the stage of retirement and contemplation. See āśrama.

Varuna   A Vedic deity; the presiding deity of the ocean.

Vedānta   (Lit., the essence or concluding part of the Vedas.) A system of philosophy mainly based upon the teachings of the Upanishads, the Bhagavad Gitā, and the *Brahma Sutras*.

Vedānta Sutras   Same as *Brahma Sutras*.

Vedas   The revealed scriptures of the Hindus, consisting of the Rig-Veda, Sāma-Veda, Yajur-Veda, and Atharva-Veda.

Vishnu (Lit., the All-Pervading Spirit.) The Preserver God; the Second Person of the Hindu Trinity, the other two being Brahmā and Śiva; also a name of the Supreme Lord.

Viśishtādvaita Qualified Non-dualistic Vedānta, a school of Vedānta founded by Rāmānuja, according to which the soul and nature are modes of Brahman, and the individual soul is a part of Brahman.

viveka Discrimination between the real and the unreal.

Vrindāvan A town on the banks of the Jumnā river, associated with Śri Krishna's childhood; also called Vrindā and Vraja.

vyādha Hunter.

Vyāsa The compiler of the Vedas, reputed author of the *Mahābhārata* and the *Brahma Sutras,* and father of Śukadeva.

Yādavas The clan of which Krishna was a member.

yajna Sacrifice.

Yajur-Veda One of the four Vedas. See Vedas.

Yaksha Mythical demigod.

Yama The king of death, a Vedic deity.

yoga Union of the individual soul and the Supreme Soul. The discipline by which such union is effected. The Yoga system of philosophy, ascribed to Patanjali, is one of the six systems of orthodox Hindu philosophy, and deals with the realization of Truth through control of the mind.

yogi One who practises yoga.

Yudhishthira The eldest of the five sons of Pāndu; one of the heroes of the *Mahābhārata.* See Pāndavas.

yuga Cycle or world period.

INDEX

INDEX